In Consciousness We Trust

In Consciousness We Trust

The Cognitive Neuroscience of Subjective Experience

Hakwan Lau

Team Leader, Laboratory for Consciousness,
RIKEN Center for Brain Science, Japan

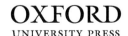

OXFORD
UNIVERSITY PRESS

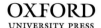

OXFORD
UNIVERSITY PRESS

Great Clarendon Street, Oxford, OX2 6DP,
United Kingdom

Oxford University Press is a department of the University of Oxford.
It furthers the University's objective of excellence in research, scholarship,
and education by publishing worldwide. Oxford is a registered trade mark of
Oxford University Press in the UK and in certain other countries

Published in the United States of America by Oxford University Press
198 Madison Avenue, New York, NY 10016, United States of America

British Library Cataloguing in Publication Data

Data available

Library of Congress Control Number: 2021947320

ISBN 978–0–19–885677–1

DOI: 10.1093/oso/9780198856771.001.0001

Printed and bound by
CPI Group (UK) Ltd, Croydon, CR0 4YY

To the truth-loving people of Hong Kong

Acknowledgments

First, I have to thank those who have taught me the most about the subject. They are my current and former students and mentees, including Brian Mansicalco, Dobromir Rahnev, Ai Koizumi, Liyan McCurdy, Yoshiaki Ko, Jorge Morale, Guillermo Solovey, Megan Peters, Vincent Taschereau-Dumouchel, Brian Odegaard, Aurelio Cortese, JD Knotts, Kiyo Miyoshi, Taylor Webb, Yujia Peng, Cody Cushing, Mouslim Cherkaoui, Raihyung Lee, Cathie So, Ben Rosenberg, and Seong Hah Cho. You'll read about some of their excellent work throughout the book.

Like Angela Clague, Matthias Michel was kind enough to read the drafts of all the chapters in this book, well before they were readable. As usual, his comments have improved the content substantially.

Of course, I also have teachers in a more formal sense. It was Chad Hansen at the University of Hong Kong, my alma mater, who first got me interested in philosophy and academia. Joe Lau at the same institution taught me how to read and write properly and planted the important seed of doubt that abstruse writing is typically anything but profound. At Oxford, Dick Passingham miraculously created a scientist out of an unruly young man.

From there, the line between mentors and friends gets blurry: Chris Frith, Joe LeDoux, Patrick Haggard, David Rosenthal, and Mitsuo Kawato taught me how to be less unwise as an academic (and as a person in general). At UCLA, Michelle Craske kindly supported my foray into clinical studies. Michele Basso and Alicia Izquierdo likewise allowed me to learn about animal models, as a late beginner.

Outside of my own affiliated institutions, Steve Fleming and Richard Brown are both good friends as well as collaborators. Our playing music *very* poorly together provided some probably pathological yet beneficial form of moral support. If nothing else, they convinced me that science, not music, is what I should focus on. Floris de Lange and Tony Ro helped me out when I needed friends to lean on in order to continue doing experiments in neuroscience. Tom Barry and Christian Chan taught me much about clinical psychology, as well as about my own home city.

Dean Mobbs and Sara Bengtsson are likewise both good friends, as well as collaborators, from the days when we all worked together in the same building in London where my theoretical ideas on consciousness first took shape. We all miss Tom Schofield very much.

There are really too many thanks to give, but I want to highlight a few people with whom I often disagree: Ned Block, Stanislas Dehaene, and Victor Lamme. It's been an utter privilege to learn directly from them. That these eminent colleagues never took intellectual arguments personally and were always willing to engage in a friendly way is what makes working in this field so special. I'm lucky enough to have also had similarly pleasant exchanges recently with Rafi Malach, Marius Usher, and Christof Koch. Although Christof and I hardly ever agree on anything, he promoted my career all the same when I started out.

The actual writing of this book started when I was on leave from UCLA, at the University of Hong Kong. While I finished the first draft back in Los Angeles, some final touches were done at the Riken Institute near Tokyo, where I currently am. I am grateful for the generous support from these three great institutions. The UCLA Library in particular has made possible for this book to be open access.

Besides some of the names already mentioned above, many other people have kindly read and commented on an earlier draft, including: Bryce Heubner, Joey Zhou, Jason Samaha, Nico Silins, Joshua Shepherd, Tony Cheng, Adrien Doerig, David Soto, Omri Raccach, Paul Dux, Grace Lindsay, and Byron Sebastian. I have also benefited from discussing drafts of this book in an undergraduate class and a graduate seminar at UCLA during the year 2021. Matthew Hin Ming Leung and Mouslim Cherkaoui both helped me with editing the final proofs.

My parents won't be reading these words, unless they are translated into Chinese. Unfortunately, I turned out to be far more irreverent than they would have liked me to be. But my skepticism toward 'authoritative' opinions came from their strong characters. This book was very much written based on that foundation.

Finally, I have to thank Kayuet Liu. We have somehow overlapped at all of the various institutions mentioned above. She is my sociology and statistics tutor, and occasional coauthor. It may be inappropriate to describe one's colleague this way, but to my mind she is also the loveliest person in the world. I hope I can get away with this because she also happens to be my spouse.

Introduction: Reality as One Sees It
I explain why we will focus on cognitive neuroscience rather than physics-centric theories.

Chapter 1: Game Plan and Definitions
Subjective experience is our focus here, though it may relate to other notions of consciousness such as wakefulness or voluntary control too. We will arbitrate between global and local theories.

Chapter 2: The Unfinished NCC Project
If we control for the key experimental confounds, the evidence is in favor of the prefrontal cortex's role in consciousness - although it may not be for the purpose of global broadcast.

Chapter 3: Hitting the Right Note
Lesions and stimulation studies are often conceptually misinterpreted or factually misrepresented. There is good evidence for the causal involvement of the prefrontal cortex in consciousness.

Chapter 4: Untouched Raw Feels?
When we don't pay attention we don't perceive much details. But our experience may be subjectively 'inflated' beyond what we actually represent in the sensory cortices; troubles for local theorists.

Chapter 5: What Good Is Consciousness?
To answer the question we need new experimental methods, beyond subliminal priming. Current evidence suggests that consciousness may not be as useful as global theories suggest.

Chapter 6: A Centrist Manifesto
Let's take stock of the findings reviewed so far. Neither global nor local theories seem right.
What are the constraints for a plausible theory? What can we learn from current AI research?

Chapter 7: Are We Alone?
We introduce the perceptual reality monitoring theory (PRM), according to which some animals may not be conscious. And yet, perhaps even a robot or computer program could be (to be revisited in Chapter 9).

Chapter 8: Making Ourselves Useful
In the social and clinical sciences, 'consciousness' often refers to our rational grasp of reality.
How is this related to the kind of consciousness we have discussed so far?

Chapter 9: What of the Hard Problem?
Subjective experiences are characterized by 'what it is like' to have them. Cognitive neuroscience can address this quality too. Metaphysical theories don't fare better, and may just hinder scientific progress.

Contents

Introduction: Reality as One Sees It   1

1. Game Plan and Definitions   13

2. The Unfinished NCC Project   33

3. Hitting the Right Note   57

4. Untouched Raw Feels?   83

5. What Good Is Consciousness?   107

6. A Centrist Manifesto   129

7. Are We Alone?   151

8. Making Ourselves Useful   175

9. What of the Hard Problem?   197

Index   221

Introduction: Reality as One Sees It

I.1 Echo Chambers

Countless eminent scholars have written on the topic of consciousness. Do we really need yet another book about it?

I am writing one because I believe that the science of consciousness is at a crossroads. On the one hand, public interest on the topic remains as high as ever. Our visibility in the media ensures that private donors recognize our challenges. At times they support us generously. Students are excited about the topic. Many are eager to join the field. In many ways, things seem to be going well.

On the other hand, it is unclear where we really stand scientifically. Outside of the field, many of our colleagues don't think much of what we do at all. Some may concede that this is just a matter of the nature of the scientific challenge we face. However, many also believe that the sheer lack of quality and rigor of the work is to blame. Unfortunately, I have to confess, sometimes I think they have a point.

Perhaps the discrepancy between the two different outlooks can be explained by two facts. The first is that scientists often vote with their feet. If they see that some field is hopeless, they may just ignore it, and focus on what they see as more tractable instead. To hear from our critics, we may need to seek them out.

I often like to hear what my 'opponents' have to say. Maybe it is in part my temperament. But I also realize—intellectual benefits aside—there are strategic reasons for engaging in this kind of conversation. The success of a scientific discipline depends not just on sheer empirical and theoretical progress. Often, acceptance by our academic neighbors matters too.

This brings me to the second reason why the negative outlook is often downplayed. Not only do our critics tend to keep their strong opinions to themselves, but those who are within the discipline are also prone to ignoring these negative comments. We often choose to live inside our own echo chambers. In part because, frankly, it doesn't seem to be good for business to emphasize too

In Consciousness We Trust. Hakwan Lau, Oxford University Press. © Hakwan Lau 2022.
DOI: 10.1093/oso/9780198856771.003.0001

much our own shortcomings or to promote them. Criticisms are also generally unpleasant to hear. But even when we aren't so shortsighted and defensive, there is this romantic feeling of going against the grain, that is pretty much shared within the community of consciousness researchers: *Historically, we know that things have been hard. But we shall ignore our critics, and soldier on. Against all the odds, we will eventually get there and prove them wrong . . .*

1.2 Romantic Ambitions

I am no stranger to this romantic feeling. After all, I have spent half of my life in this somewhat controversial field.

In college, I read Dave Chalmers' *Conscious Mind* (1996)). Like the grunge and alternative rock music that was popular around the time of its publication, the book shook my world. Besides the refreshingly clean arguments, I distinctly remember how *cool* it was, that a rising star of a young scholar expressed so beautifully his heartfelt frustration at the many attempts to reduce our subjective experiences down to some physical processes. Those attempts can sometimes lead to "elegant theories," I recall Chalmers wrote, *but the problem does not go away.*

Don't get me wrong—I was, and still am a cognitivist, in the sense that, I believe the best way to understand the brain is to think of it as a biologically instantiated computer. Concepts from electrical engineering and computer science have proven to be great analogies, if not straightforward theoretical constructs, for understanding how the brain functions. That's our bread and butter.

But there is one problem sticking out like a sore thumb. Machines just don't seem to *feel* anything, however sophisticated they are at processing signals. So conscious perception cannot just *be* a matter of processing signals because there are these unexplained *raw feels*. There is *something it is like* seeing the color red. It's more than just picking up some wavelength values of incoming lights. Explaining how these subjective experiences come about is what Chalmers called the Hard Problem, and it does sound like one indeed.

This was, to my impressionable young mind then, on par with Gödel's application of devilishly clever logical analysis to show that mathematics can never be complete (Smullyan 1998). By taking the hard problem of consciousness seriously, we are recognizing that cognitive neuroscience may too be *incomplete*.

Somehow this did not prevent me from going to graduate school to study more cognitive neuroscience. There, many of my fellow students and

professors alike would snicker at the silliness of my lofty philosophical obses-
sions. We *are* cognitive neuroscientists. Why worry about problems that we
can't solve anyway? If a problem is decidedly so 'hard,' why not find something
more rewarding and tractable to *do*? Being a good scientist is to be realistic
about what we can or cannot do.

But, I thought, the first step toward solving a problem is to recognize that
there is one. My fellow students and professors were probably too conventional and conservative. *I shall ignore them, and soldier on.* I was particularly
encouraged when I learned that the Nobel laureate Francis Crick suggested
we put the sign "Consciousness NOW" in our labs and offices. If such great
minds as Crick thought that the time was ripe for attack (1994), we had to be
onto something.

Who knows? Perhaps decades later, we would find that we have done all we
can within the limits of cognitive neuroscience, and *lo and behold*, indeed, we
cannot solve the hard problem. We may need something more. Something
like a *revolution*. In that sense, we are working on the edges where things may
eventually break down in unpredictable ways. Indeed, they say that we may
even have to revise the very foundation of physics to accommodate the occurrence of subjective experiences (Chalmers 1996). There just seems to be
no room for such subjective phenomena within the ordinary language of objective science.

Like the opening power chords of Kurt Cobain's song *Smells Like Teen
Spirit*, these possibilities seemed so intoxicatingly exciting to my ju-
venile self.

But later I found out that I was wrong. Not because young people shouldn't
dream big. But because I was fundamentally misguided about some historical facts.

1.3 A Convoluted History

Like many currently active researchers in the field, I used to think that the scientific studies of consciousness were somehow "revived" in the 1990s. Or perhaps it really all started around then, with only feeble activity here and there
before that was very much suppressed in the heydays of behaviorism. That
narrative was so prevalent that, even when I was a graduate student at Oxford,
where Larry Weiskrantz was still active in research, I just thought he must be
an anomaly.

Weiskrantz coined the term *blindsight*, which refers to the phenomenon
that people with specific brain damage can show behavioral signs of successful

visual information processing, such as being able to guess the identity of a visual stimulus, all without having conscious visual experience. Much of the work demonstrating the phenomenon was done in the 1970s and 1980s (Weiskrantz 1986).

And then, of course, in neuroscience textbooks, we all know about the amnesic patient HM, studied by Brenda Milner and others. Patient HM can form new nonconscious memories in the form of motor learning. What seemed to be most problematic was that he was unable to form new conscious memories of events as they occurred to him (what is also called episodic memory). Most of these details were documented as early as in the 1950s (Scoville and Milner 1957). So perhaps, another anomaly?

Yet another classic line of work that is no doubt relevant to consciousness is on split-brain patients. After having the major connections between the two hemispheres surgically severed, information presented to the right hemisphere alone cannot be verbalized. Michael Gazzaniga and colleagues have shown that some of these patients showed behavioral signs of being able to process and act on such information. However, much of that behavior seems opaque to conscious introspection. Again, many of these studies were done well before the 1990s (LeDoux, Wilson, and Gazzaniga 1979).

Far from anomalies—except in the sense of being extraordinarily influential—Weiskrantz, Milner, and Gazzaniga are all household names in neuropsychology. Their groundbreaking discoveries are taught today in undergraduate classrooms around the globe. Gazzaniga himself coined the term *cognitive neuroscience*. He is also often considered to be one of the founding grandmasters of the field. His PhD advisor with whom he did some of the split-brain patient work together was the Nobel laureate Roger Sperry. Sperry too wrote on the topic of consciousness (1965, 1969)—well before the 1990s.

Outside of neuroscience, important work has been done in other areas of psychology too. To give just a few examples, in cognitive psychology, Tim Shallice developed elegant models of attention and conscious control of behavior (1972, 1978). In social psychology, Leon Festinger's work on cognitive dissonance continues to be extremely influential to this date (1957). There, it was proposed that subjects have a need to reduce our internal conflicts. Resolving these conflicts can at times lead to rather unexpected behavior and change of attitudes. All of which seems to happen largely nonconsciously. In psychophysics, that is the quantitative analysis of perceptual behavior, Pierce and Jastrow have written on the relationship between subjective awareness and confidence ratings as early as over a century ago (Peirce and Jastrow 1885).

So, my romanticized vision about the science of consciousness turned out to be based on some serious misunderstanding. I thought studying consciousness was akin to some sort of martyrdom. We were preparing for a revolution, to break away from an unforgiving scientific tradition in which there was no place for consciousness—not before the 1990s anyway. But that was just not true.

I.4 The "Mindless" Approach

So what happened in the 1990s, exactly? What kind of revolutions were we really talking about? It would be unfair to deny the hugely positive impact of what took place then. In a series of meetings started in the early 1990s in the city of Tucson, Arizona, some of the truly great scientists of our times gathered together and plotted strategies for attacking this age-old problem of consciousness. Besides Crick, another Nobel laureate, Gerald Edelman, was also there. The Wolf Prize winner Sir Roger Penrose (now a Nobel laureate too) also attended. In those meetings a research agenda for a generation was set, and stars were born.

It's not entirely clear how it went, but somehow a misleading narrative also emerged that the modern science of consciousness started more or less right there. There's some truth to the fact that consciousness science as a relatively *organized* activity really flourished from those meetings. Inspired by the Tucson meetings, a couple of journals dedicated to the topic started, another meeting spun off: the Association of the Scientific Studies of Consciousness (ASSC) was created. But it is not true that those were the first-ever academic conferences on consciousness (LeDoux, Michel, and Lau 2020).

Instead, what really happened was that a rich and ongoing history of studies of consciousness in cognitive neuroscience and psychology were somewhat sidelined. Replacing it was a newfound obsession for physics and other natural science disciplines. The creation of ASSC restored that balance to some degree. But back in Tucson, the biannual meetings continue to attract media and public attention. The popular impression is clear: our agenda is to unlock the mystery of consciousness, and to understand our place in nature. It is a challenge for all of the natural sciences. In fact, it is one of the few remaining scientific frontiers that truly matter. Or so the narrative goes.

Perhaps this focus on the "bigger picture" isn't so bad. As yet another Nobel laureate, Rutherford, famously said, in science, there is really only physics (Birks 1962)—*the rest is just stamp collecting.*

But I have never found Rutherford's comment convincing. Good for him that he won the Nobel for chemistry. But as soon as one moves from chemistry to biology, it is well-known that lawlike reductions to physics fail (Fodor 1974; Kitcher 1984). It is all very well that water is H_2O, and hydrogen and oxygen can be defined precisely in terms of atoms, protons, electrons, and things like that. But just how does one give physical, lawlike definitions of biological functions such as digestion or reproduction?

This is not to say that biological functions are not instantiated by purely physical stuff. They are. The problem is there are no laws or equations that you can conveniently write down, in fundamental physical terms, to parsimoniously describe these functions. These functions can be realized by many different forms of physical substrates. A gut can be replaced by a functional equivalent made of rather different materials. Good luck finding fundamental physical laws about digestion. Even if one finds some equations that can fit some current data, more or less, treating them as "laws" of nature is a totally different matter.

So when I heard someone like the physicist Max Tegmark (2015) argue that consciousness may be ultimately about how the physical parts of an organism are arranged together, as if this too can be described in some simple clever equations, I just felt … maybe the 1990s were in part to blame. Perhaps the infamous "decade of the brain" misled some of us to think that understanding the "software" of the brain—that is, that fluffy thing called the "mind"—isn't as cool and impressive as going straight to the hardware. But that would be getting ahead of ourselves. If one ever wants to write down some equations at the level of physics to distinguish between a conscious and an unconscious brain, how about we first try writing down some equations to distinguish between a computer sending emails properly, versus an annoying computer which, upon having the "send" button clicked, just silently saves the drafts in the outbox without ever sending them? Can one really ignore the nitty-gritties of software, algorithms, and the like, and directly derive physical first principles there?

1.5 Before Newton

Some colleagues may feel that I'm just being too pessimistic. After all, in physics, great things have been achieved through theorizing in the abstract. Had Einstein shied away from his bold attempts at deriving the first principles, the world we live in today would be utterly different. Few would describe what

Einstein did as "reverse engineering" of a specific, messy system. It was just pure theory, on the most general and foundational level.

But what if Einstein was born in a different place and time, such as in ancient Greece, where thinkers also wondered about the universe? There, armchair theorizing seems not to have done nearly as much good. One may wonder if that was because Newton and Leibniz had not yet invented the beautiful tools of calculus for them. Perhaps the Greek thinkers did not make more progress because they lacked the precise language of advanced mathematics?

But the Newtonian laws of motion were not just written down out of sheer analytical genius. The foundation of mechanics was also built on rigorous empiricism. The laws were accepted, sometimes rather grudgingly by Newton's critics, only because they were *empirically* verified over and over again (McMullin 2001). Although these laws ultimately turn out to be incomplete (as things get extremely small or large), they give theoretical physicists a solid platform on which further derivations and inferences can be made. Had Newton got the basic facts flat wrong, no amount of elegant equations could have saved him.

Today, our mathematics are far more advanced than in the days of Newton's. But, in the science of consciousness, we are still very far from having all the relevant basic facts. It would take some profound misunderstanding of the scientific method for one to think that some such foundational laws can be derived from the sheer comfort of the armchair.

1.6 Responsible Revolutionary Planning

Despite my misgivings, I do not mean to say that ambitious universal theories can never offer any insight for understanding consciousness. The problem is, once we get past all the rigorous-looking abstruse mathematical details, often we find that the underlying assumptions are shaky and controversial (Sloman 1992; Cerullo 2015; Bayne 2018; Pautz 2019). Sometimes, the theorists commit simple logical fallacies and contradict their very own definitions (Lau and Michel 2019a). Or they make neurophysiological and anatomical claims that just seem not quite right by textbook standards (Odegaard, Knight, and Lau 2017).

These are not intrinsic problems of theoretically ambitious approaches; the concerned theorists do not *have* to neglect these details. But the problem is they often do. I worry this reflects some important sociological aspects of the sciences that are too often overlooked (Lau and Michel 2019b).

In consciousness research there has been an unduly heavy focus on personal glory and stardom. Rarely in any area of neuroscience do we think that there are these age-old puzzles, waiting to be solved by some destined genius. That's because science is generally about progress. As we work on a problem, we aim to achieve a better understanding, not to close the book forever. Of course, game-changing discoveries do happen occasionally, but only the most foolish narcissists would *expect* them to happen *in one's own hands*. In the event of such a windfall, one should be grateful for the groundwork already done by those before us.

This is not to say that we must focus on incremental empirical progress alone. The conceptual issues about consciousness are intriguing and are why many of us are here in the first place. But as Thomas Kuhn famously pointed out (1962), scientific revolutions require undeniable evidence—so undeniable as to force us to accept the inadequacy of our current paradigm. This threshold to revolution is ultimately determined by *the scientific community*.

Imagine we have to tell our colleagues in cognitive neuroscience that their approach is decidedly incomplete. Don't we have to first earn their respect? How convincing would that be if they just don't think we are even capable of telling rigorous science from utter nonsense?

And if we are so ambitious as to hope that one day we can tell the physicists to rewrite their textbooks, so as to accommodate our subject matter at their foundational level ... how would we look if our colleagues next door point out that we are just flat wrong in the most elementary biological facts, while we are making these grandiose proposals?

Revolutions are exciting. But we don't call for them without the necessary ammunition. I fear though, sometimes we aim too high without being able to actually deliver. Amid all the media glory, we neglect that the *academic* reputation and longevity of the field matters. Meanwhile, career and public funding prospects remain grim for young scientists studying consciousness, especially in the United States (Michel et al. 2018, 2019). Sometimes I wonder: are we so deluded to think that the next generation doesn't matter because we think we can start and finish the said revolution ourselves right here?

I.7 Between the Vanilla and the Metaphysical

So throughout this book I will advocate for a conservative—or perhaps even *boring*—empirical approach for studying consciousness. We shall remain interested in the deeper philosophical issues, but getting the empirical facts right shall ever be our first priority.

This approach is conventional in the sense that it basically is just run-of-the-mill cognitive neuroscience these days. To those already familiar with the literature, one may wonder if this means that current major theories like the global workspace theory already suffice (Dehaene 2014)? The answer is: no. We will introduce some of these views in the next chapter, and expose their inadequacies through Chapters 2–6. That motivates a novel, alternative view.

Our overall goal here is to find mechanistic explanations for consciousness, borrowing concepts from electrical engineering and computer science. We try to figure out what may be the relevant computational processes. We infer what these may be, based on a combination of modeling and observing currently measurable neural activity in the brain. We use standard tools like neuroimaging, invasive neuronal recording, and electrical and magnetic stimulations. We ask questions like: What type of activity in what brain region may be important? What kind of cognitive functions are reflected by this activity?

We may not be able to explain everything we need to in the end. But let's see. At least we *first* give it a fair shot before we rush into something more radical. My hope is to convince you that, boring as all this may sound, much light can be shed on consciousness this way.

One may ask though, if the goal is to fully integrate with the modern standards of cognitive neuroscience, why use the term *consciousness* at all? Why not replace it with something less controversial, perhaps already existing in the literature, like, for example, working memory, attention, metacognition, and perception?

The answer is that even if we stay within the language of modern cognitive neuroscience, there is ample room for defining a notion of consciousness (i.e., of subjective experience) that is distinct from these other related concepts. Take for example perception. As we mentioned earlier, blindsight patients have certain visual perceptual capacities. What is lacking is a reported sense of subjective visual experience (Weiskrantz 1986). So, perception-like processes are not always conscious. Understanding perception alone would not be enough to understand consciousness. We also need to understand the mechanisms that render these processes sometimes conscious, and sometimes not.

And likewise, throughout the book we will argue that although consciousness is highly related to mechanisms such as metacognition, working memory, and attention, for example, it is really a distinct phenomenon.

But even if there is a distinct phenomenon, why *call* it consciousness? Why not sidestep the whole historical baggage and create a more precise technical term instead? Trouble is, I'm not sure this kind of eliminativism has ever really worked. No doubt *water* is a somewhat vague term. It is not as precise as H_2O.

But chemists don't tell us to stop saying *water*. Even if they did, I wonder if it would have mattered.

Whether we like it or not, the term *consciousness* is used in many disciplines, from psychiatry to political theory. This is what many people care about. The very notion of consciousness has its roots in the social sciences as well as in mental health research. Often, there are real, meaningful questions to be asked, regarding the role consciousness plays in these contexts. But the current answers often seem murky, not because they have to be. Rather, I fear that we have somehow failed our duty. Between worrying too much about lofty metaphysical problems, or overreacting to the other "vanilla," eliminativist extreme, we simply have not done our job. We have made it sound like no serious scientific claims can be made about the brain mechanisms for consciousness. But the concept isn't going away.

It is time to do our part.

1.8 Chapter Conclusions

Consciousness is the mechanism by which we derive our subjective sense of reality. Ironically, within the consciousness research community, different colleagues don't always see the same reality at all. This division may be particularly salient between the two sides of the Atlantic (Michel et al. 2018, 2019). For various reasons, the cognitive neuroscience of consciousness is doing somewhat better in Europe. But it is unclear how the field can truly flourish if it remains primarily a regional activity. On the Pacific front, we face yet another set of challenges; will the science of consciousness in countries like Japan, China, and Australia become more like what happens in the United States or Europe? Or will it become something totally different altogether?

I started by pointing out that the field is at a crossroads. So what options are we facing? Obviously, one way to go is to do nothing. Judging by how things have gone in the past decade, things may well become increasingly esoteric and theoretically indulgent, especially in the United States. Many may think that's fine. We will probably not run out of "big ideas" any time soon. The popular media, together with a few wealthy private donors, will probably continue to like us all the same.

Alternatively, we can make a case for why it may not be such a bad idea to be a little more aligned with common scientific standards. After all, if we aren't so misguided about the history of the field, we realize that much of the most meaningful work on consciousness has been done this way, rather than in some unrealistic revolutionary spirit. Perhaps, with some luck, we can eventually break into the scientific mainstream.

As such, one can also say that the point of this chapter is just to lower expectations. To avoid disappointment, perhaps I should warn the reader there will not be any elegant formula allowing you to derive that your teacup is exactly 0.00000247% as conscious as your cat, or anything of equivalent mind-bending proportions. In all likelihood, your metaphysical worldviews will be left unchanged.

But does this mean that we will have nothing meaningful to say about the *hard problem* after all? I hope not. I think we will. Let's find out. But to do so, I'm afraid you have to read to the end.

References

Bayne T. On the axiomatic foundations of the integrated information theory of consciousness. *Neurosci Conscious* 2018;niy007.

Birks JB. *Rutherford at Manchester*. Heywood, 1962.

Cerullo MA. The problem with phi: A critique of integrated information theory. *PLoS Comput Biol* 2015;**11**(9):e1004286.

Chalmers DJ. *The Conscious Mind: In Search of a Fundamental Theory*. Oxford Paperbacks, 1996.

Crick F. *The Astonishing Hypothesis: The Scientific Search for the Soul*. Pocket Books, 1994.

Dehaene S. *Consciousness and the Brain: Deciphering How the Brain Codes Our Thoughts*. Penguin, 2014.

Festinger L. *A Theory of Cognitive Dissonance*. Stanford University Press, 1957.

Fodor J. Special sciences (or: The disunity of science as a working hypothesis). *Synthese* 1974;**28**(2):395–410.

Kitcher P. 1953 and all that: A tale of two sciences. *Philos Rev* 1984;**93**:335–373.

Kuhn TS. *The Structure of Scientific Revolutions*. University of Chicago Press, 1962, DOI: 10.7208/chicago/9780226458106.001.0001.

Lau H, Michel M. *On the Dangers of Conflating Strong and Weak Versions of a Theory of Consciousness*. Philosophy and the Mind Sciences, 2019a, DOI: 10.31234/osf.io/hjp3s.

Lau H, Michel M. *A Socio-Historical Take on the Meta-Problem of Consciousness*. Imprint Academic, 2019b, DOI: 10.31234/osf.io/ut8zq.

LeDoux JE, Michel M, Lau H. A little history goes a long way toward understanding why we study consciousness the way we do today. *Proc Natl Acad Sci USA* 2020;**117**:6976–6984.

LeDoux JE, Wilson DH, Gazzaniga MS. Beyond commissurotomy: Clues to consciousness. *Neuropsychology* 1979;**2**:543–554.

McMullin E. The impact of Newton's Principia on the philosophy of science. *Philos Sci* 2001;**68**:279–310.

Michel M, Beck D, Block N et al. Opportunities and challenges for a maturing science of consciousness. *Nat Hum Behav* 2019;**3**:104–107.

Michel M, Fleming SM, Lau H et al. An informal internet survey on the current state of consciousness science. *Front Psychol* 2018;**9**:2134.

Odegaard B, Knight RT, Lau H. Should a few null findings falsify prefrontal theories of conscious perception? *J Neurosci* 2017;**37**:9593–9602.

Pautz A. What is the integrated information theory of consciousness? *J Conscious Stud* 2019;**26**:188–215.

Peirce CD, Jastrow J. On small differences in sensation. *Biogr Mem Natl Acad Sci* 1885;**3**:73–83.

Scoville WB, Milner B. Loss of recent memory after bilateral hippocampal lesions. *J Neurol Neurosurg Psychiatry* 1957;**20**:11–21.

Shallice T. Dual functions of consciousness. *Psychol Rev* 1972;**79**:383–393.

Shallice T. The dominant action system: An information-processing approach to consciousness. *The Stream of Consciousness* 1978:117–157.

Sloman A. The emperor's real mind: Review of Roger Penrose's the emperor's new mind: Concerning computers, minds and the laws of physics. *Artif Intell* 1992;**56**:355–396.

Smullyan R. Gödel's incompleteness theorems. In: Goble L, ed. *The Blackwell Guide to Philosophical Logic*. John Wiley and Sons Ltd; 2001:72–89.

Sperry RW. Brain bisection and mechanisms of consciousness. In: John C. Eccles, ed. Brain and Conscious Experience. Springer Verlag; 1965:298–313.

Sperry RW. A modified concept of consciousness. *Psychol Rev* 1969;**76**:532–536.

Tegmark M. Consciousness as a state of matter. *Chaos Solitons Fractals* 2015;**76**:238–270.

Weiskrantz L. *Blindsight: A Case Study and Implications*. Oxford University Press, 1986.

1
Game Plan and Definitions

1.1 An Overshadowed Literature

In the last chapter, I said that my point was to lower expectations. But the wise reader may see that it could backfire too. After all, it has been famously remarked that nothing worth reading has ever been written on consciousness (Sutherland 1989). It may be easy to be conventional and boring, but can any degree of scientific rigor ever be achieved on the topic, really?

Truth is, nothing would please me more than if I ended up inadvertently attracting a bandit of fierce critics to methodically tear my views apart. As a field, we can benefit from having more critics.

Thankfully, though, I do not have to defend the cognitive neuroscience of consciousness all by myself. Over the past couple of decades, a community of active researchers dedicated to doing solid work on the topic has emerged. This work is sometimes overshadowed by more "exciting," revolutionary proposals, especially in the popular media. So I take the opportunity to review the relevant literature here.

However, even within this group of researchers who identify themselves as cognitive neuroscientists, ideas and theories abound. Having many ideas is often a good thing, but they are only useful to the extent that we have enough decisive experiments and quality data to arbitrate between them. Unfortunately, I cannot say that this is currently the case, in part for reasons explained in the last chapter. As such, any attempt at providing a comprehensive review risks producing nothing but a list of "who said what when." I am tempted to do so for diplomatic reasons. But ultimately that would not be particularly useful for the reader. So let me take you through a shortcut instead.

1.2 Global Theories

According to global theories of consciousness, subjective experiences arise when the relevant information is broadcast to many regions in the brain. The philosopher Dan Dennett once likened the phenomenon to "fame in the brain" (1991).

In Consciousness We Trust. Hakwan Lau, Oxford University Press. © Hakwan Lau 2022.
DOI: 10.1093/oso/9780198856771.003.0002

The idea traces back to Bernard Baars's global workspace theory (1989), according to which the brain has specialized "modules," including those for language, long-term memory, motor control, and perception in specific modalities. These modules are informationally encapsulated (Fodor 1983). They mostly mind their own businesses. But now and then, they need to communicate with each other. They can do so by setting up a direct one-to-one contact, which need not reflect consciousness. For example, when you play your favorite fast-paced ball game, your motor control system is probably very much connected to your visual perceptual system (assuming you are any good at it, and you're in the zone). The relevant reflexes are so fast that they may not be fully conscious.

But most of the time, when we are not in such highly rehearsed situations, how the modules access, store, and coordinate information among themselves is not so clear. When you see a person on the street, you don't automatically engage the motor system to reflexively act. Instead, there is probably some central system, in which the relevant information is stored for all modules to access and edit. This central system is likened to a workspace, a hub for exchange of information. According to the theory, information becomes conscious in the brain if and only if it enters this workspace. So when you consciously see someone on the street, your visual perception module puts that information in the workspace for other modules to access. This allows you to talk about it, act on it, remember it, check if it is coherent with what you hear, and what you smell, for example. That is what consciousness involves: the global broadcast and central executive control of information.

Stanislas Dehaene put these ideas into the context of known neuroanatomy and physiology (2014). According to what he calls the global neuronal workspace theory, the relevant mechanisms for consciousness critically depend on activity in the prefrontal and parietal cortices (Figure 1.1), where neurons have long-range connections with many other regions in the brain. This view is supported by ample empirical evidence, as we will see in the next chapters.

Overall, global theories of consciousness, and their very many variants, are endorsed by numerous active research groups (Cohen et al. 2012; Joglekar et al. 2018; Mashour et al. 2020).

1.3 Local Theories

In contrast, we also have local theories, according to which subjective experiences happen when the right kind of neural activity occurs in the relevant sensory modality. Take vision as an example. According to local theories, we

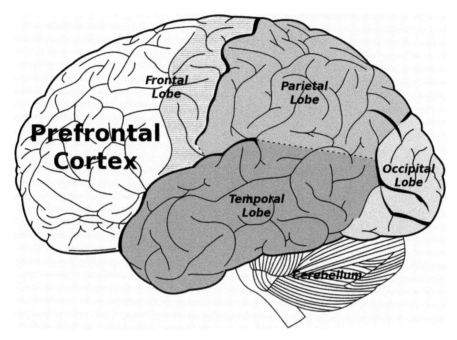

Figure 1.1 Global theories suggest that prefrontal and parietal areas in the brain are causally important for subjective experiences to arise

consciously see something when and only when there is the right kind of activity in the visual cortex. The rest of the brain isn't really critically involved.

Like global theories, there are many flavors here. To some, what constitutes the right kind of activity within the visual cortex depends on the specific brain regions where the activity happens. For example, according to authors like Rafi Malach (Fisch et al. 2009, 2011) and Stephan Macknik and Susana Martinez-Conde (2008), the key regions for visual consciousness are the extrastriate areas, which are visual cortical areas outside of the primary visual cortex (also known as striate cortex or V1). Ultimately, this may also depend on the special visual feature in question; motion and color may depend on different regions (Zeki 2001).

What may also be critical is the dynamics, or the temporal profile, of the activity. For example, Victor Lamme (2003, 2006) argued that what is critical for conscious experience to arise is recurrent activity, first supported by a feedforward wave, for example, from V1 to an extrastriate area (e.g., middle temporal area, MT), and then followed by feedback to V1 (Figure 1.2).

As in many other subfields of research on the neuroscience of perception, studies of vision tend to dominate somewhat. There may be historical reasons for this (Hubel and Wiesel 2004; LeDoux, Michel, and Lau 2020), as well as

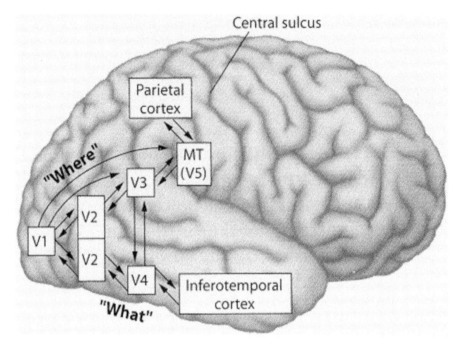

Figure 1.2 Local theories suggest that subjective visual experiences critically depend on specific activity within the visual areas in the brain

considerations of experimental logistics. Some find this unfortunate, and they may be right about that (Smith 2017; Barwich 2020). But regardless, one can think of equivalent ideas in other modalities too. For example, in hearing and touch, there are primary sensory areas in the cortex as well. According to Lamme, feedback to these early cortical areas may also be important. The hope is that once visual consciousness is better understood, the principles derived from this research may generalize more or less to other modalities.

Again, just like global theories, local theories have ample empirical support, as we will see in the next few chapters.

1.4 Theoretical Goal Posts

I mentioned that I would take you through the literature via a shortcut. Here is how: the global and local theories are polar opposites, representing two extreme ends of a theoretical spectrum. By contrasting these two views, we can quickly cover a lot of ground.

As such, the two views are to be treated as somewhat hypothetical guiding points. Like goal posts in a ball game, they work best if they are static. That is to say, to serve this purpose, I will at times treat each of the family of theories more or less as a singular, stable view. In reality this is often not quite true. Not only are there different versions of global theories, but Dehaene himself has also changed his position on some details over the years (Naccache and Dehaene 2001; Dehaene 2014; King, Pescetelli, and Dehaene 2016), for example. Likewise, Lamme seems not to always insist that feedback to V1 is important; other forms of recurrent activity may also do the job (2016), perhaps.

So there is a risk of misrepresenting these authors. I will try to be as clear as possible in ascribing specific ideas to individual researchers. Beyond that, I have to count on them, along with many other important theorists who are not mentioned in this framework, for understanding. As indicated earlier, my goal here is not to provide a detailed review of all the theories. Rather, it is to summarize the landscape in a gist to orient ourselves. As in any good map, we sacrifice some details. So for each side, we will focus on a representative, prototypical version of the theory. When I say "global theories" or "local theories" I refer to these generic views. They are inspired by the specific authors mentioned in the last sections, but do not necessarily reflect their latest thinking. Once we know the rough orientations, specific versions of their latest views can be better articulated and understood. The rest of the chapter, I hope, will convince the reader of the usefulness of this framework.

Perhaps some theories will fall outside of the spectrum, as they may be considered more extreme than local theories. Not only do they refuse to identify consciousness with some cognitive functions like global theories do, perhaps even the physical substrate proposed may be more abstract than the commonly measured neural activity in a brain region. The substrate may have nothing to do with neurons per se. Perhaps what matters is some general physical properties in the relevant structure. But these are mostly physics-centric theories that are not entirely compatible with the modern language of cognitive neuroscience. As we will see (in Chapters 6, 8, and 9), to the extent that local theories fail, these views will also be in trouble. So we don't need to worry about them too much here.

1.5 The Fine Art of Definitions

Even at this level of convenient abstraction, a tricky conceptual problem arises as we compare the global and local views. Perhaps the two views are different only because they adopt different definitions of consciousness? So they may just be talking past each other?

So far, I have deferred precisely defining the very phenomenon we are after. Some readers may find this odd. Perhaps this should have been done at the very beginning of the book. But issues regarding definitions are sometimes treacherous. They are often better handled after some warming up.

To illustrate the problem, let's change the topic for a moment, to consider the definition of *fish*. In kindergarten, I recall getting upset when my teacher insisted that dolphins are not fish. *But they look like fish, and they swim in the ocean.* Just why was my teacher "correct," and I "wrong"? Turns out, Aristotle actually also classified dolphins as a kind of fish; the kind with lungs (Romero 2012). So one may be tempted to say that my disagreement with my kindergarten teacher was nothing but *a matter of definitions.* She just defined *fish* in a way different from the way I did. We just talked past each other. With Aristotle on my side too, obviously I wasn't so wrong?

While we certainly disagreed on the definition, it doesn't mean that's the end of the argument. Some definitions are better than others. But how to evaluate this is often not so straightforward. In the case of *fish*, modern biologists have decided that it is better to say dolphins are mammals instead. In part, that's because dolphins don't lay eggs, and they don't have scales. But that's hardly the end of the story either. Just why is laying eggs more important as a criterion for being a fish than being able to swim in the ocean? Why doesn't how it looks matter the most?

In the end, biologists decided that a certain taxonomy is better for their purposes. It helps to highlight some facts that are important to them. By adopting their taxonomy, things hang better overall with other pieces of knowledge considered by them to be relevant and established: for example, evolution.

The moral of this story is that definitions are often a matter of ongoing negotiation. At times, they are almost like political debates. They are political in the sense that some definitions serve certain purposes better. But as soon as we talk about purpose, we need to ask: *whose* purpose? Maybe classifying dolphins as mammals fits better with the phylogenetic understanding of the animal kingdom, which in turn allows biologists to make some reliable scientific inductions based on the relevant categorical labels. But my kindergarten self didn't care about that. To my mind then, how it looked was more important. All I needed to know was what belonged to the ocean, rather than the sky or land. I suppose some poets and painters may be on my side too. It may matter little to them what biologists think. But of course, in the end, the biologists had their ways. Collectively, society agreed that they produce more useful knowledge than I did. The poor kid in kindergarten lost the political battle.

1.6 Access Versus Phenomenal

Back to the problem of consciousness. It is a similar situation. To decide what definitions to adopt, we first need to think about what is the relevant purpose: in other words, what is the problem we are trying to solve? This is why, although we didn't talk about definitions, in the introduction, we introduced the "Hard Problem" (Chalmers 1996), that is the challenge of explaining subjective experience in purely mechanistic terms. From there, it should be clear that *if* our goal is to have something meaningful to say about the Hard Problem, what should primarily concern us here would be subjective experience.

By subjective experience, I mean the "raw feels" associated with certain mental processes. Some mental processes are nonconscious, in the sense that they don't feel like anything. We sometimes say there is *"nothing it is like"* to be in those relevant mental states. In fact we mostly don't even realize when such processes are taking place. But some other mental processes are conscious. To consciously see certain things, for example, the color red, involves a certain feel. We sometimes say, there is *"something it is like"* to see red (Nagel 1989). That subjective aspect of the perceptual process is what we are concerned with here. Our overall scientific goal here is to map out the differences between conscious and unconscious mental processes—that is, to figure out why some mental processes are associated with subjective experiences and others aren't.

For subjective experience, other terms I use synonymously include *conscious experience, qualitative experience, subjective feel, raw feel, phenomenology, phenomenality, phenomenal quality, phenomenal experience, phenomenal consciousness,* and *conscious awareness.* They all mean the same thing. For precision I really should stick to one term only. However, for variety and flow, I sometimes sacrifice absolute precision. Whenever unspecified, *consciousness* refers to this "default" notion of subjective experience, rather than some other notions such as wakefulness or control, which we will discuss in the next two sections.

The philosopher Ned Block famously distinguished phenomenal consciousness from another notion called access consciousness (1995). Access consciousness happens when a relevant piece of information in the brain becomes available for cognition, or for the rational control of action.

Now, this may look like a way to dissolve the debate between global and local theories before it even starts. One could perhaps argue that global theories are really just about access consciousness. And local theories are about phenomenal consciousness. Because these are two different definitions, they are just talking past each other. Of course, the rational control of action may require the global broadcast of relevant information. But maybe this has nothing to do with how subjective experiences come about. So both theories may be right, without conflicting with each other.

However, this way of thinking assumes that access consciousness may be totally dissociable from phenomenal consciousness. Two definitions can be conceptually different, and yet, in reality, they may just come down to the very same things. For example, *water* can be defined as colorless liquid at room temperature, of certain viscosity, lacking flavor and odor. Or, it can be defined in terms of its precise chemical constituent, H_2O. But they may just end up referring to the very same substance, in this world at least.

Likewise for access versus phenomenal consciousness. Conceptually they sound different enough. But are they really distinct phenomena in the brain? Can we ever have one without the other, entirely? What exactly is subjective experience without the relevant information impacting our reasoning and rational control of action in *any* way? If we truly *feel* pain, how can it not affect our cognition and decision to act at all? If we consciously *see* the color red, how can it not bear any influence on our thinking that there is something red in front of us?

I shall refrain from assuming one way or the other here, regarding the possible dissociation between phenomenal consciousness and access. Chapter 4 will address this as a challenging empirical question. The point here is to say: just because others have defined a notion of consciousness that is allegedly distinct from access does not mean that we have to *accept* the definition. Maybe phenomenal consciousness turns out to always come with at least some degree of access.

Regardless of the empirical outcome, the scientific community may well also come to agree that it is just more *useful* to focus on a notion of subjective experience that isn't entirely distinct from access. There may be some aspects of subjective experience that are distinct from access, but maybe the community would decide that it is really not of our interest. Those who insist on a definition otherwise may end up being like the poor kid in kindergarten who insists that dolphins are fish. How this plays out will depend on our ongoing investigation and negotiation. As we shall see, this will not be trivial at all.

So for now, we will not assume that global and local theories concern distinct phenomena. Although some global theorists sometimes say that their views are about access consciousness (Dehaene et al. 2014), they do not really refer to a kind of consciousness lacking in subjective experience entirely. Subjective experience is what we all really care about, global and local theorists alike. Because the two views are ultimately about the same phenomenon—at least as construed here—they are substantively different theoretical positions.

1.7 Coma Patients and Experimental Confounders

By focusing on subjective experience, we see why some other notions of consciousness are at once highly relevant, and yet not quite useful enough for our scientific purposes.

In everyday life, of course, the common usage of the term *consciousness* mostly has to do with wakefulness: as in, when we have too much (alcohol) to drink, we pass out, and lose consciousness. Patients suffering from traumatic brain injury, such as from car accidents, may also lose consciousness, or even go into a prolonged coma. Likewise, global anesthesia is meant to put people into nonconscious states. Typically we use this notion of consciousness to refer to the individual, or a state that the individual is in. Subjective experiences, on the other hand, are typically associated with specific mental processes occurring in an individual, like the process of visually perceiving something.

But this common notion of consciousness as applied to the general state of the individual is not unrelated to subjective experiences either. When we are unconscious, as in being entirely unawake and unresponsive, we typically cannot enjoy subjective experiences—unless we are in dreams. So *consciousness* in this sense may be defined as having the capacity to have subjective experiences.

Besides having to deal with the exceptional case of dreams, one trouble is that when one is awake with the capacity to have subjective experiences, one is also capable of doing many other things. When one is conscious rather than unconscious, one can remember things, talk about them, think about them, and produce complex behavior. Overall, our brains are presumably processing a lot more information in much more sophisticated ways than when we are unconscious. This is probably true in dreams too, even though we tend not to act out our behavior physically there.

So, if the goal is to scientifically understand the mechanisms for subjective experience, comparing the brain activity of someone conscious against someone who is in a coma would not be so useful. There will be many confounding factors, in the sense that besides having subjective experiences, many other things also differ between the two cases. So let's say if we find that there is more activity in one part of the brain in the conscious over the unconscious individual, we will not know for sure whether this is specifically due to the occurrence of subjective experiences or something else that is also lacking in the unconscious individual (as mentioned previously).

This is why in this book we will not focus too much on coma patients, the state of being in an epileptic seizure, or anesthesia. Understanding these cases has important practical implications. Wonderful experiments have been done on them. But they will not be our empirical starting points, because for our specific purpose of understanding the basic mechanisms for subjective experiences, they suffer from having too many experimental confounders.

This issue of experimental confounders is of central importance. Yet it is often overlooked, even by experts. We will come back to this issue again and again.

1.8 Purposeful Behavior and Experimental Confounders (Again)

Another notion of consciousness, which applies to both the individual, as well as specific mental processes, is purposeful control. When one is fully awake and conscious, one can consciously control one's actions. When one is in a deep coma, one produces no action at all. But in between, there is what Adrian Owen calls the "gray zone" (2019). In such states of semiconsciousness—which can also be achieved by drinking heavily but not *too* heavily to completely pass out—one makes actions that are somewhat routine, as if they aren't under conscious control.

This same notion of consciousness applies to specific mental processes too. Some processes, such as the decision to book a plane ticket through a particular airline to go to a specific destination, tend to come with some sense of volitional control. The individual tends to feel ownership and responsibility for the results of these processes. We say that these decisions are made consciously. Some other processes, on the other hand, may happen relatively quickly and reflexively, such as our attempts to regain balance after almost tripping over a rock on the street. Often, we do not feel that these processes are entirely up to our purposeful control, and we say that the corresponding actions are not fully consciously made.

This notion of consciousness, as in the control of purposeful behavior, may be related to subjective experiences too. Specifically, when applied to mental processes rather than the individual, when we say a process is conscious, it comes with the subjective experience of volitional control, or what is sometimes called a sense of agency. Also, for a process to be conscious in the sense of purposeful control, it is possible that its inputs need to be consciously experienced. That is, when we make consciously controlled actions, we may not actively take into account nonconscious information: that is, information conveyed by mental processes not associated with any subjective experience. At least, it is likely that in making conscious actions we rely more on conscious rather than nonconscious information.

We will address some of these issues in Chapters 5 and 8. The reasons for deferring them for later is again related to experimental confounders. Conscious and nonconscious actions may well differ in terms of their relationship with subjective experiences, including the very conscious experience of volition. But conscious actions also tend to be more complex, and the corresponding information processes tend to be more powerful and sophisticated. So, by comparing typical conscious and nonconscious actions, we risk having too many experimental confounders, and this would limit what we can learn about the specific underlying processes.

The reader may notice that what is discussed regarding confounders here and in the previous section is somewhat against the spirit of what we discussed in Section 1.6, when we argued that phenomenal and access consciousness may not be empirically dissociated. There, we pointed out that we cannot just define *subjective experience* as having nothing to do with informational access. But if subjective experience turns out to be empirically always linked to such informational access, then how can we consider the latter to be a confounder?

An analogy may help to illustrate this delicate point: in comparing tall people versus short people, we do not say that the length of one's bones is a confounder. That is because being tall *is* to have longer bones. It makes no sense to say, we match the length of all the bones of two individuals, so as to specifically look at their difference in physical height. Likewise, if subjective experience is the very same thing as having global information access—which we suggested in Section 1.6 *may* be the case—then there would be no point in controlling for the latter as a confounder either.

So this issue of confounders is very thorny indeed. Much as we like to think of controlling for confounders as a simple matter of scientific hygiene, the conceptual issues involved are often far from straightforward. Specifically, if we define subjective experience as always having to do with sophisticated information processing, allowing rational access and control, we are automatically loading the dice in favor of global theories. If we define *subjective experience* as having decidedly nothing to do with these sophisticated information processes, we are likewise tilting the table in favor of local theories. This is why we cannot assume one way or the other from the outset. Nor can we end the debate by saying it is just a matter of definitions, followed by a shrug. These issues must be carefully examined on a case-by-case basis, depending on the experiments and phenomena concerned. Each time we set out to control for a confounder, we need to ask: Is this meaningful? Or is it begging the question?

Is it even possible in principle? Ultimately, the experiments need to be convincing, and, unfortunately, plausibility is not always a hard-and-fast objective matter.

1.9 Five Key Issues

Having now cleared the ground about the various conceptual issues and definitions, we can outline the key issues on which we will arbitrate between the global and local theories. As explained earlier, it is best to start with the more straightforward issues and move on from there to the more speculative ones. So the ordering matters here.

The first issue concerns the relevant neural mechanisms, also sometimes called the neural correlates of consciousness (NCC). This may be the most obvious issue because the global and local theories are more or less defined in terms of the NCC. For local theories, the NCC is the activity within the sensory regions of the modality concerned. For global theories, activity outside of the sensory regions is involved. The NCC includes activity in what is sometimes called the "association areas," in the prefrontal and parietal cortices, where neuronal coding doesn't seem to be specific to a single sensory modality.

The second issue concerns the richness of subjective experience. Global theories hold that the content of subjective experience is gated by attentional mechanisms, which is to say, by and large, we only consciously perceive what we are attending to. Therefore, subjective experience is relatively sparse. Outside of attentional focus we do not consciously experience all the details. On the other hand, local theories hold that subjective experience is relatively rich, because capacity limits owing to late-stage processing (e.g., prefrontal broadcast) do not really matter for consciousness. Our subjective experiences are as rich as what early sensory processing can afford.

The third issue is about the functions of consciousness. What are the cognitive advantages of conscious processes, compared to nonconscious processes? Global theories identify consciousness with a powerful cognitive mechanism, the central workspace. Without entering this workspace, the relevant information cannot exercise certain important cognitive functions; for, otherwise, we would not need to have this workspace in the first place. Local theories, on the other hand, make no such commitments. Without having the right kind of activity in the early sensory regions, the information can travel all the way to downstream, late-stage mechanisms without ever becoming conscious. Which is to say, nonconscious processing can be very powerful too. So consciousness may not come with substantive cognitive advantages.

The fourth issue concerns whether other creatures are conscious like we are. That is, we will finally consider the notion of consciousness as applied to an individual. Is consciousness a uniquely human phenomenon? What about very young children? What about primates and smaller animals? On global theories, consciousness ultimately is a higher cognitive mechanism, which some animals may lack. Or at least, like in young children, their global broadcast mechanisms may not be as developed as ours, so even if they were conscious, their capacity for having subjective experiences may be relatively limited. For local theories, once again, these late-stage mechanisms don't matter. Children and some animals may well not have very advanced and developed prefrontal cortices, but this should not limit their conscious experiences.

The fifth issue is similarly controversial, if not more so. It concerns whether machines and robots can ever be conscious. As in the last one, answers to this fifth issue will necessarily be somewhat speculative. If consciousness ultimately is a cognitive mechanism, aligned with what global theories say, one should be able to build the functional equivalent in robots. But this seems to imply that consciousness may already be possible in some current machines, which may seem counterintuitive. Local theories, on the other hand, can hold that the key is having the right kind of biological substrate. This blocks the possibility of consciousness in current robots but offers no principled account as to what makes a biological substrate special.

To summarize, these are the five main questions that we will tackle: 1) Is the NCC global? 2) Is subjective experience sparse rather than rich? 3) Is consciousness important for higher cognitive functions? 4) Is consciousness somewhat limited in young children and primitive animals? 5) Is machine consciousness ever possible? Global theories say *yes* to these five questions. Local theories say *no* to them all. This is why we consider the two views as polar extremes.

1.10 The Need for a Coherent Synthesis

There are of course many other questions one can ask about consciousness. Why focus on these five?

One reason is that I myself actually struggle to come up with other questions of as much contemporary and historical significance as these five, which are at the same time also somewhat tractable at the moment. In part, that's because these questions are logically connected, so there is a factor of synergy.

As we address the first issue regarding the NCC (Chapters 2 and 3), it helps to constrain the answers for the second issue of richness (Chapter 4). That's because if the NCC depends on activity in higher cortical areas (e.g., the prefrontal cortex), then the capacity limits of the relevant late-stage processes may apply. To anticipate, based on the presently available evidence, I will indeed argue that the prefrontal cortex is constitutively involved in the generation of subjective experiences. But the causal role of this involvement may not be global broadcast. As such, it poses some limit to the actual richness of subjective experience. But perhaps it can support an "inflated" sense of richness. That is, the rich details may not be represented as such because the brain may not have the capacity to do so properly. But some mechanisms may exist to fool ourselves, subjectively, that we have these rich details.

So the conscious phenomenology is somewhat rich, but not *really*. This kind of intermediate answer will be a recurring motif. Overall, the empirical evidence is not so kind to either the global or local views.

Likewise, the third issue of functions (Chapter 5) depends somewhat on our take on the first two issues. This is so, especially, because there are tricky methodological issues preventing a clear, direct empirical answer thus far. Given the nature of prefrontal involvement in consciousness, we may expect some functions to be uniquely tied to subjective experiences. But I will argue that these functions are not so general as global theories imply; many high cognitive functions are influenced and controlled by nonconscious information. But consciousness may provide an advantage to some specific functions, such as metacognition and inhibition of some specific process.

As to the fourth and fifth issues, of animals and machine consciousness, they can only be resolved with the help of a theoretical perspective. The earlier "empirical" chapters will be summarized in Chapter 6, which will provide constraints about what a plausible theory should look like. From there, we will outline a view (Chapters 7–9) according to which our brain mechanisms for consciousness may be shared by some mammals. However, some other animals may lack these mechanisms. And yet, in principle, we can build these mechanisms into robots and machines, and make them conscious too. (That is to say, philosophically, I'm a functionalist, as I'll explain in Chapters 6–9.)

Throughout, I will try to be fair to review others' empirical work when they are relevant and decisive. I will no doubt miss many important experiments still, out of sheer ignorance and forgetfulness. The reader will also find that I am evidently biased in favor of reviewing my own work. This is my book after all. So I hope that's okay.

1.11 Theoretical Upshot

I anticipate that some readers will want to jump straight to Chapter 6 for the summary of the earlier empirical reviews. In a way, the chapter was written exactly for this purpose; I appreciate that some people may not have the time to read books from cover to cover. But I do not recommend skipping the earlier chapters, even for the philosophers. The answers are important. But new findings may come along and change what we know. What will remain useful are the concepts and rationale behind the arguments and interpretations.

For similar reasons, I hesitate to give a soundbite summary of my theoretical views here. If this book has a single take-home message, it is that genuine scientific progress requires us to care about the details. My primary purpose here is to review and synthesize a rather large body of literature, not to profess a narrow viewpoint. But I've also been told that readers tend not to go beyond the first chapters of any book, unless they are sufficiently enticed. So here is my best attempt: Based on the discussion of empirical findings, it should become clear that subjective experience is not entirely disconnected from cognition. There are good motivations for not confounding the two, and the global theorists might have been too quick to assume that consciousness is just a form of strong and stable information processing. All the same, even in experiments in which all reasonable controls are carried out, subjective experiences are somehow linked to at least some degree of impact on the cognitive mechanisms in the prefrontal cortex (Chapters 2 and 3). These mechanisms are also needed to account for the subjective richness of experience (Chapter 4), as well as some empirically observed functional advantages of conscious processing (Chapter 5).

As such, a good theory needs to account for this subtle link between consciousness and cognition, without contradicting empirical data. Introspectively, most authors seem to agree that subjective experiences have this so-called here-and-now quality. They present themselves as reflecting the state of the world, or some ongoings in our bodies, *at the current moment*. This seems to be an indispensable property of conscious experiences. When we are in pain, it is difficult not to worry that something bad is happening to us at the relevant bodily location. Even if we are ultimately convinced that nothing really is wrong physically (it may be a "psychic" or illusory pain), it is difficult to shake off the strong tendency to think about that. This potential tendency seems somewhat intrinsic to the experience.

I will therefore propose in Chapter 7 that a conscious perceptual experience requires not just a representation of the sensory content but also a further representation to the effect that the sensory representation is reflecting the state of the world right now. That is why a perceptual experience is generally not confused with a memory representation of the same content, which we know does not reflect the world *right now*. The experience of a vivid memory recall is supported by a different kind of further representation. But when this further representation is missing altogether, there should be no subjective experience. This explains why sometimes sensory representations alone do not lead to conscious experiences at all (as in conditions like blindsight or aphantasia).

So this further representation is necessary for conscious experiences to occur. We can call this a higher-order representation. It is generated automatically by a *subpersonal* process. That is, we don't have to think hard to come up with this higher-order representation. It's not a thought in that sense. This higher-order representation serves as a tag or label indicating the suitable epistemic status of the sensory representation, and functions as a gating mechanism to route the relevant sensory information for further cognitive processing. Because such further processing is only a potential consequence, but not a constitutive part of the subjective experience, this sets my view apart from global theories. In other words, consciousness is neither cognition nor metacognition. It is the mechanistic interface right between perception and cognition. Current evidence suggests that such higher-order mechanisms likely reside within the mammalian prefrontal cortex, where the functions of perceptual metacognition are also carried out; I will explain why there is such overlap at the physical implementation level.

The local theorist may reject this notion of consciousness, in favor of a definition concerning purely "raw" experiences, with no constitutive connection to cognition whatsoever. Besides empirical evidence, I will survey some broad theoretical considerations, from the clinical and social sciences (Chapter 8). It is also in this context that we can best understand the nature of emotions, culture, rationality, and free will. Ultimately, the local theorists could insist on using whatever definitions they so prefer. But some definitions will not allow us to speak to these important issues of historical and practical interests. One runs the risk of defining oneself into an obscure corner of isolation—just like that poor kid in the kindergarten mentioned in Section 1.5.

To be fair, likewise, we also need to make sure that our theory does not ignore some local theorists' primary concerns about the subjective character or phenomenal quality of experiences. These issues may have been given less weight within the clinical and social sciences, but philosophers have debated about them for centuries. I will argue in Chapter 9 that our theory can account for the qualitative aspects of experience too.

In philosophy, we often say that there is "something it is like" to be a conscious agent enjoying some specific subjective experiences. I take it that the qualitative aspects of an experience can be understood in terms of its similarity relations with respect to all other possible experiences. The complexity of these exact relations accounts for why it may seem so hard to express the subjective quality of a conscious experience in words. But once these relations are "known," the subjective quality is fully determined. This is all there is to having subjective phenomenology. Red looks the way it does because it is subjectively more similar to pink than to blue, more similar to orange than to silver, and so on (with *all* the relevant similarity relations spelled out in exact terms). It looks *redder* than everything else.

I will further argue that because of the way the mammalian sensory cortices are organized, perceptual signals in the brain are spatially "analog" in a specific sense. I will outline the computational advantages for having these representations organized this way. These explain how we likely evolved to have this functional feature of our brains. Given this analog nature, when the higher-order mechanisms discussed herein correctly address a sensory representation, the relevant similarity relations are all implicitly "known." So when a sensory representation becomes conscious, not only do we have the tendency to think that its content reflects the state of the world right now, also determined is *what it is like* to have the relevant experience—in terms of how subjectively similar it is with respect to all other possible experiences. I submit that this addresses the Hard Problem, better than prominent alternative views.

1.12 Chapter Summary

Here we introduced the local and global views, as useful theoretical goalposts. Between the two extremes, there lies a spectrum on which an empirically plausible middle ground can hopefully be found. A plan is set out for reviewing the literature in the coming chapters, going through the five issues of 1) the NCC; 2) richness of experience; 3) functions of consciousness; 4) consciousness in young children and animals; and 5) the possibility of machine consciousness. These will allow us to arbitrate between the global and local views. To anticipate, we will find that neither position works. But we will learn much from the process of understanding their limitations, respectively. Striking a balance is the key.

We also went through four different notions of consciousness: 1) subjective experience, 2) access consciousness, 3) consciousness as the state an individual is in, and 4) consciousness as purposeful control. Subjective experience is what we will focus on, but it does not mean that the other notions are entirely distinct. They may empirically turn out to be very much related. We will find out.

Above all, we warned ourselves of some treacherous conceptual issues, regarding definitions and confounders. They are anything but straightforward. If not careful, we may inadvertently tilt the table rather unfairly in favor of one side of the spectrum before the competition even begins.

As in the introduction, here we spent a fair bit of time explaining why certain things will not be discussed much further. The next chapter is where the positive scientific journey really begins.

References

Baars BJ. *A Cognitive Theory of Consciousness.* Cambridge University Press, 1989.

Barwich AS. *Smellosophy: What the Nose Tells the Mind.* Harvard University Press, 2020.

Block N. On a confusion about a function of consciousness. *Behav Brain Sci* 1995;**18**:227–247.

Chalmers DJ. *The Conscious Mind: In Search of a Fundamental Theory.* Oxford Paperbacks, 1996.

Cohen MA, Cavanagh P, Chun MM et al. The attentional requirements of consciousness. *Trends Cogn Sci* 2012;**16**:411–417.

Dehaene S. *Consciousness and the Brain: Deciphering How the Brain Codes Our Thoughts.* Penguin, 2014.

Dehaene S, Charles L, King J-R et al. Toward a computational theory of conscious processing. *Curr Opin Neurobiol* 2014;**25**:76–84.

Dennett DC. *Consciousness Explained.* Little Brown, 1991.

Fisch L, Privman E, Ramot M et al. Neural "ignition": Enhanced activation linked to perceptual awareness in human ventral stream visual cortex. *Neuron* 2009;**64**:562–574.

Fodor JA. *The Modularity of Mind.* MIT Press, 1983. https://doi.org/10.7551/mitpress/4737.001.0001.

Hubel DH, Wiesel TN. *Brain and Visual Perception: The Story of a 25-Year Collaboration.* Oxford University Press, 2004.

Joglekar MR, Mejias JF, Yang GR et al. Inter-areal balanced amplification enhances signal propagation in a large-scale circuit model of the primate cortex. *Neuron* 2018;**98**:222–234.e8.

King J-R, Pescetelli N, Dehaene S. Brain mechanisms underlying the brief maintenance of seen and unseen sensory information. *Neuron* 2016;**92**:1122–1134.

Lamme V. *The Crack of Dawn: Perceptual Functions and Neural Mechanisms That Mark the Transition from Unconscious Processing to Conscious Vision*. In: Metzinger T, Windt JM, eds. Open MIND, 22(T). MIND Group, 2016.

Lamme VAF. Why visual attention and awareness are different. *Trends Cogn Sci* 2003;**7**:12–18.

Lamme VAF. Towards a true neural stance on consciousness. *Trends Cogn Sci* 2006;**10**:494–501.

LeDoux JE, Michel M, Lau H. A little history goes a long way toward understanding why we study consciousness the way we do today. *Proc Natl Acad Sci U S A* 2020;**117**:6976–6984.

Macknik SL, Martinez-Conde S. The role of feedback in visual masking and visual processing. *Adv Cogn Psychol* 2008;**3**:125–152.

Malach R. Conscious perception and the frontal lobes: Comment on Lau and Rosenthal. *Trends Cogn Sci* 2011;**15**:507; author reply 508–509.

Mashour GA, Roelfsema P, Changeux J-P et al. Conscious processing and the global neuronal workspace hypothesis. *Neuron* 2020;**105**:776–798.

Naccache L, Dehaene S. Unconscious semantic priming extends to novel unseen stimuli. *Cognition* 2001;**80**:215–229.

Nagel T. *The View From Nowhere*. Oxford University Press, 1989.

Owen A. Into the grey zone: Detecting covert conscious awareness in behaviourally non-responsive individuals. *J Neurol Sci* 2019;**405**:2.

Romero A. When whales became mammals: The scientific journey of Cetaceans from fish to mammals in the history of science. In A Romero and EO Keith (eds), *New Approaches to the Study of Marine Mammals*. InTechOpen, 2012. https://www.intechopen.com/chapters/40763.

Smith BC. Human olfaction, crossmodal perception, and consciousness. *Chem Senses* 2017;**42**:793–795.

Sutherland NS. *The International Dictionary of Psychology*. Crossroad Publishing Company, 1989.

Zeki S. Localization and globalization in conscious vision. *Annu Rev Neurosci* 2001;**24**:57–86.

2

The Unfinished NCC Project

2.1 Derailment

Some of my colleagues who are familiar with the scientific literature will probably snicker as they skim through the opening chapters. All that high-sounding long-windedness to state the obvious. Isn't an empirical approach grounded in cognitive neuroscience what we have always been doing?

It is true that this approach is really nothing new. In recent times, we sometimes say we are trying to find the neural correlates of consciousness (NCC). This so-called NCC project started in the 1990s. But as with the whole idea of a "revival" of consciousness science, there too is a long and often neglected history well before that (Michel 2019; LeDoux, Michel, and Lau 2020).

Not knowing our history is a problem beyond pedantic concerns of scholarship, because we are prone to repeating the same mistakes. The trouble is that some conceptual issues are hard to avoid, even when we think we are focusing on "straight-ahead" empirical studies of consciousness. In recent years, in fact, we have seen many of these same problems creep up again (Michel and Lau 2020). Amid some exciting calls for *moving on* to more theoretically adventurous endeavors, there is a worry that the empirical project itself could well be derailed. The purpose of this chapter—as well as the next—is to set us back on the right path.

2.2 Mere Correlates?

In cognitive neuroscience, we look for neural mechanisms for psychological phenomena. Rarely do we say we are merely looking for *correlates*. When we say a certain neuronal circuit provides a mechanism for a psychological phenomenon, we mean they are causally or constitutively relevant (Craver 2007). For example, certain neuronal firing patterns in the motor cortex lead to specific patterns of muscular movements. Some other neuronal firing patterns in the hippocampus make possible the formation of certain memories.

In Consciousness We Trust. Hakwan Lau, Oxford University Press. © Hakwan Lau 2022.
DOI: 10.1093/oso/9780198856771.003.0003

Understanding these neuronal circuits is supposed to provide mechanistic accounts of the phenomena.

But for consciousness, things are trickier. Some may think that such mechanistic explanations won't ever be possible. Perhaps certain neural pattern is just *one and the same* as the conscious experience itself (Place 1956). This identity view is somewhat different from the causal view, because logically speaking, a thing cannot cause itself. But to say we are looking for the neural identities or identifiers for consciousness may be too strong; not everyone is happy with the identity view either. This can lead to endless debates about metaphysics. In order to sidestep the issues, the more neutral term of *correlates* was adopted.

But correlates is a very weak notion. As they often say, correlations need not imply causation. Things that aren't directly causally connected may well be correlated. For example, people's consumption of ice cream and use of swimming pools are correlated over the year. But that is not because eating ice cream makes people swim more, or the other way around. Both are just caused by another factor: the heat in the summer. So likewise, many neural activity patterns will be correlated with consciousness, but they too may be neither causally nor constitutively relevant. Perhaps they just reflect the state of being awake, or the ability to produce complex behavior, which isn't quite the same as subjective experiences.

2.3 Necessity and Sufficiency

So there have been some attempts to finesse the definition of the NCC, by borrowing the precise language of necessity and sufficiency from logic and philosophy. The NCC is sometimes said to be the minimally sufficient conditions for a subjective experience to occur, given certain background conditions (e.g., oxygen in the blood or an intact brain stem; Chalmers 2000). This rules out some distal, indirect correlates. That is, if this NCC occurs, we must have the relevant subjective experience (given the background conditions).

The trouble is that we scientists are actually not very good at using this language. Worse still, we often overlook the complexity involved (Miller 2014; Michel and Lau 2020). To appreciate this, one can try explaining the following to their colleagues in neuroscience or cognitive psychology: so the engine of my car is what really drives it. It is both necessary and sufficient for the car to move around.

So far, so good? Shockingly, many would think so, especially if you mention it in passing without warning. But of course, if we think carefully, the engine is not necessary for the car to move around at all. Without the engine, we can push the car. Or maybe it's a hybrid so there is also an electric motor. So even though the engine is the primary causal mechanism, it is not necessary, strictly speaking. Nor is it sufficient. If I leave the engine intact, but take off the wheels, the car wouldn't move around.

The moral here is to not to say we scientists can't think logically. Most of us can, if we pay attention to what the terms "necessity" and "sufficiency" *really* mean. But this is precisely the point: we must always pay attention. Specifically, there are two caveats to bear in mind: First, abolishing the primary causal mechanism (e.g., the engine) may not always abolish the relevant function. This is true for sufficient conditions in general; they aren't irreplaceable. The specification in the NCC definition that they need to be *minimally* sufficient helps to rule out that we are not including within the NCC a large set of mutually redundant conditions. This is to say, we are hoping to home in on the barebones. This may give the ring that these are the "minimal *necessities*," and perhaps this is why scientists confuse themselves at times. But barebones aren't strictly necessary in the logical sense. Just because we do not include redundancy in our definition of the NCC does not mean there's no redundancy in the brain. These barebones (minimally sufficient conditions) could well be replaced by something else—perhaps something clumsier, less minimalist, and less efficient—which may end up doing a similar job. This is a tricky point that we will revisit again in the next chapter.

Second, abolishing some peripheral mechanisms (e.g., the wheels or the gas tank) may well abolish the relevant function, even when the primary causal mechanism itself is intact. In terms of the NCC definition of minimal sufficiency, that's because other background conditions may be necessary. The clause about background conditions exists for good reasons.

As we will see, these two caveats are often neglected, sometimes by some of the original proponents of the NCC definition themselves (Michel and Lau 2020). So even if we don't like to think of the NCC as a causal mechanism (e.g., because of metaphysical considerations), it is often helpful to think of it *almost as if* it is one, just so as to remind ourselves of the two caveats above. It is easier to think clearly this way, in terms of mechanisms, rather than in terms of necessary and sufficient conditions.

2.4 Blindsight & the Primary Visual Cortex

As we mentioned briefly in the introduction, blindsight is the neurological condition in which subjective experience in vision is selectively impaired (Weiskrantz 1997). These patients deny that they consciously see, but when pressed, they can "guess" the identity of simple visual stimuli in front of them correctly. Because blindsight is traditionally found in patients with restricted lesions to the primary visual cortex (V1), it has been suggested that V1 is a good candidate for the visual NCC (Lamme 2001, 2003).

This is supported by some studies involving subjects from the general population too. In these studies, transcranial magnetic stimulation is applied to V1. Under the right stimulation parameters, this disrupts the ongoing neural activity in the area, creating a temporary "virtual lesion" effect. This abolished perceptions which would otherwise be conscious (Pascual-Leone and Walsh 2001; Boyer, Harrison, and Ro 2005; Ro et al. 2010).

On the face of it, these findings may seem to support the local view of consciousness introduced in Chapter 1. But, of course, this is where the second caveat from the last section comes into play. How do we know that a normally functioning V1 is not just a normally required background condition? Most of the visual information from the eyes enters the cerebral cortex through V1. So lesioning V1 may be a bit like cutting off the tube from the gas tank to the engine. It may abolish the relevant functions, but V1 may not be the engine itself (Silvanto 2015).

Turns out, by stimulating other visual areas, researchers could induce conscious visual experience in a blindsight patient without V1 too (Mazzi, Savazzi, and Silvanto 2019). There have also been reports of patients with damage to the visual cortex who experienced vivid hallucinations (discussed in Lau and Brown 2019), or that they can voluntarily engage in conscious mental imagery (Bridge et al. 2012). So the engine does look like it could be elsewhere.

2.5 Content Mismatch in Early Visual Areas

So, lesions alone, real or virtual, may not tell us the full story. Fortunately, there are also many studies measuring neural activity in V1. Some of these studies showed that activity in V1 was in fact correlated with many aspects of the subjective experience of seeing (Tong 2003). But this is not always true.

For example, it is known that we are rather poor at identifying which eyeball is the origin of certain visual information (Schwarzkopf, Schindler, and Rees 2010). If I flash some light briefly to one of your eyes in a controlled laboratory setting, you will most likely see the light but will not be so good at pinpointing which of the two eyeballs received the stimulation. And yet, some cells within V1 are highly sensitive to this information. Many neurons are mainly driven by stimulation to one eye but not the other.

This may be fine for local theorists. They can say that not all activity in V1 is part of the NCC. Some activity in V1 may reflect information of which we are not consciously aware. But still, the visual NCC can be within a subset of activity in V1. Also, some local theorists may say that the NCC is not within V1. Extrastriate areas (Macknik and Martinez-Conde 2008; Fisch et al. 2009; Malach 2011), and/or their feedback projections back to V1 (Lamme 2001, 2003), are perhaps more important.

However, using imaging methods that measure the overall population activity of brain regions, others have found strong nonconscious effects in V1 and beyond. That is, population activity within most visual areas seems to be able to distinguish between stimuli that subjectively look identical (e.g., Jiang, Zhou, and He 2007; Zhang et al. 2012; Huang et al. 2020). One common idea in these studies is to use various "tricks" from vision psychophysics to create a visual illusion of some sort. So the physical stimulus may be presented in a certain way, but subjectively it looks a different way. The question is whether activity in early visual areas tracks the physical stimulus or the subjective percept, under such illusory conditions when the physical and subjective come apart.

One such experiment was based on the double-drift illusion (Liu et al. 2019). A Gabor patch is an abstract stimulus often used by vision scientists. It looks like what is shown in Figure 2.1. When the pattern within the Gabor patch shifts locally, sometimes we mistake the entire patch to be drifting (i.e., relocating) sideways, even when it really isn't. Liu et al. (2019) contains links to video demonstrations of the illusion.

This experiment was conducted using functional magnetic resonance imaging (fMRI), where subjects' brain activity was indirectly measured (via local blood oxygenation changes). By looking at the fine-grained spatial pattern of activity in different brain regions—a method also known as multivoxel pattern analysis (MVPA)—the researchers first trained an algorithm (also called a decoder) to classify the motion based on actual physical drifts (i.e., relocation, not local pattern shifts). After the researchers identified that these spatial patterns of activity represented normal drift signals, they tested whether similar patterns occur during the illusory drifts. They found that this was not the case for any of the visual areas tested. So the visual areas seem to represent the physical movement of the stimulus, not the subjective percept.

In another study also using fMRI, the researchers manipulated the subjectively perceived duration of a simple visual stimulus using sinusoidal gratings (stimuli somewhat similar to a Gabor patch). Again by inducing local pattern shifting within the stimulus, they shortened the perceived stimulus duration subjectively. However, under the illusion, they found that in early visual areas,

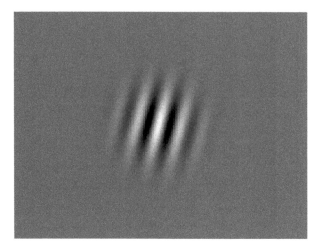

Figure 2.1 A Gabor patch

the signal correlated with the actual physical duration, rather than the sub-jectively perceived duration (Binetti et al. 2020).

Just for yet another example using a different neuroimaging method, magnetoencephalography (MEG), others and I have scanned subjects while they judged the brightness of some disks. By exploiting another illusion, called the temporal context effect (Eagleman, Jacobson, and Sejnowski 2004), we changed the subjective brightness of a disk, without changing its physical brightness. Typically, we expect certain patterns of activity within the early visual cortex to correlate positively with brightness. But instead, we found the opposite relationship (Zhou et al. 2020).

As an aside, this was a form of adversarial collaboration, perhaps one of the firsts in the field. Although I was more sympathetic to something akin to the global view when I was planning the study, the data were analyzed mainly by researchers in support of a local view (Sandberg et al. 2013). Together, we tried to find correlates in the early visual areas. We just couldn't. Or, we could say we did, but they turned out to be the opposite as expected.

Overall, the temporal aspects of early visual activities may also be problem-atic if they are treated as candidates for the NCC. Because early visual activities reflect specific perceptual content, the straightforward localist interpretation is that as a certain subjective experience occurs, visual activities should reflect the relevant content at that moment. However, conscious experience takes some time to be fully determined, whereas early visual processes are relatively fast. Our awareness of a stimulus presented at time t is known to depend on stimuli presented up a fraction of a second later. Therefore, Michel and Doerig (2021) argued that early visual correlates probably do not have the right time scale to match our conscious experiences.

Relatedly, when two similar stimuli are presented in close succession, the second stimulus is known to elicit weaker activity in the early sensory regions. This phenomenon is sometimes called repetition suppression (Gotts, Chow, and Martin 2012). However, subjectively, we don't tend to perceive the second stimulus as being substantially weaker. Again, this suggests that without some downstream calibration mechanisms, early sensory activities alone are unlikely to always match the content of subjective experiences.

2.6 Distal Cause versus the "Engine" Itself

I do not mean to say that subjective experiences don't correlate with early visual activities at all. Apparently they do, in many studies (Tong 2003). But one may also expect a certain publication bias is at play: vision scientists tend to start with the hypothesis that such correlates can be found within the visual areas, and when they are not, the study may be considered a failure, and accordingly the negative findings may not be reported.

For the sake of argument, let us grant the local theorists that overall, there are likely many more cases where the subjective percept correlates with early visual activity. There is still a problem, though, if this correlation breaks down in a good number of minority cases. This may suggest that the early visual areas are just a distal cause of subjective experience, a bit like the retina itself. Of course retinal activity correlates with features of what we see *most* of the time—but not all the time, which is why we generally don't think of the retina as part of the NCC. So the cases mentioned in the last section, where the subjective percept and early visual activity come apart, may be critical.

There is of course an issue of sensitivity in the measurements. Using neuroimaging, sometimes we fail to observe certain signals. But they may be observable using more sensitive methods like invasive single cell recording. However, in both of the fMRI experiments mentioned (Liu et al. 2019; Binetti et al. 2020), when the researchers could not find the expected correlates within the visual areas, such correlates are found elsewhere (e.g., in the prefrontal cortex)—where sensitivity for neuroimaging measurements is typically weaker (Bhandari, Gagne, and Badre 2018). Therefore, the negative findings in the visual areas seem not to be due to measurement limitations alone.

2.7 Fronto-Parietal Network

So under the double-drift and subjective temporal duration illusions, the subjective percept seems to correlate well with activity in the prefrontal and

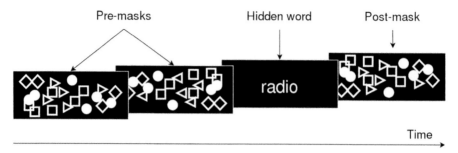

Figure 2.2 The visual masking technique

Reproduced with permission from Dehaene, S., Naccache, L., Cohen, L. et al. (2001). Cerebral mechanisms of word masking and unconscious repetition priming. *Nat Neurosci,* 4, 752–758. https://doi.org/10.1038/89551

parietal areas (Liu et al. 2019; Binetti et al. 2020). This is congruent with a very large body of work accumulated over decades, showing the importance of activity from these higher regions in consciousness (Rees, Kreiman, and Koch 2002; Dehaene 2014; Dehaene, Lau, and Kouider 2017; Odegaard, Knight, and Lau 2017; LeDoux, Michel, and Lau 2020).

In many of these studies, the researchers compared a "conscious" condition where the subjects saw the stimulus (sometimes called the "target"), with a "nonconscious" condition where the subjects did not see the stimulus. Comparing these conditions typically reveals robust and widespread activations in the prefrontal and parietal areas, that is, higher activity for the conscious condition.

For example, Dehaene et al. (2001) compared words that subjects were able to consciously see and recognize, against the same stimuli embedded in some distracting visual patterns, called forward (pre) and backward (post) visual "masks," which made the words invisible and unrecognizable (Figure 2.2). This comparison revealed some differences in the visual areas too. But the difference was more striking in the prefrontal and parietal areas. Under the nonconscious condition, the activity in these areas was near baseline level, as if these regions were engaged exclusively under conscious perception.

2.8 Stimulus Confounder

Global theorists, including Dehaene himself, have taken the results mentioned in Section 2.7 to support their views (Dehaene 2014; Dehaene, Lau, and Kouider 2017). But it could be argued that there was a stimulus confounder in these studies. That is, while the conscious and nonconscious conditions differed in perception, the stimuli presented also differed. So the observed activity could be driven by the physical stimulus difference rather than reflecting subjective experience itself.

There are two common ways to deal with this stimulus confounder. One is to present a stimulus at an intermediate intensity. We can use psychophysical methods to titrate the stimulus so that it will be presented at around detection threshold. At this level, sometimes subjects see it consciously, and sometimes they don't. Then after the experiment, we can sort out the "consciously seen" trials versus the "nonconscious" trials and make the comparison. This way the comparison will involve stimuli presented at the same physical intensity. Many studies employed this strategy and found evidence in support of the global view (e.g., Carmel, Lavie, and Rees 2006).

Another way is to make use of the phenomenon of bistable percepts, in which a static physical stimulus may give rise to different subjective percepts over time. One popular example is binocular rivalry (Blake, Brascamp, and Heeger 2014); see Figure 2.3. This occurs when we present different images to the two different eyes, using laboratory optical instruments. When set up correctly, most subjects will not see a static fusion of both images. Instead, they see one image for a few seconds, and then spontaneously a perceptual switch occurs, after which they see the other image for a few seconds, and then switch again, back and forth and so on. Typically, these perceptual shifts occur automatically, as in, beyond the subject's volitional control. When the subject sees one image but not the other, we say that the seen image is in dominance and the other image is under suppression.

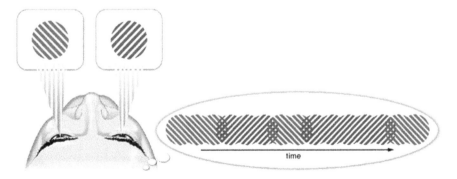

Figure 2.3 Binocular rivalry

Reproduced under a Creative Commons Attribution-NonCommercial 3.0 Unported (CC BY-NC 3.0) from Dieter, K., C., and Tadin, D. (2011). Understanding attentional modulation of binocular rivalry: a framework based on biased competition. *Front. Hum. Neurosci*, 5:155. doi: 10.3389/fnhum.2011.00155

Using binocular rivalry, many studies have found evidence in support of the global view too. With fMRI, many researchers have found an increase in activity in the prefrontal and parietal areas when the perceptual switch occurs (Rees, Kreiman, and Koch 2002). Using methods at a higher resolution, such as invasive neuronal or local field potential recording, it has been reported that activity in these areas can reflect the image in perceptual dominance too (Panagiotaropoulos et al. 2012). Let's say, for a hypothetical example, that the two images in rivalry are left-tilted and right-tilted line patterns, respectively, as shown in Figure 2.3. The logic of these studies is that we can first identify activity in the prefrontal cortex reflecting one image, say the left-tilted line patterns. When the subject sees the left-tilted line pattern, this activity would show an increase. When the same left-tilted line pattern is under suppression, that is when the subject sees the other pattern (the right-tilted lines), this activity would be low.

But others have taken similar studies as support for the local view because early visual activity also tracks the shifts in the subjective percept under binocular rivalry. Although the suppressed image tends to be reflected by some activity in the early visual areas too, the level of activity tends to be lower than that for the dominant image. This difference is in fact rather salient in the visual cortex. However, as we will see next, they may not reflect changes in subjective experience per se.

2.9 The Trickiest Confounder of All

Binocular rivalry elegantly addresses the problem of stimulus confounder. Accordingly, among consciousness researchers it is commonly regarded as an extremely important experimental tool. However, experts on binocular rivalry have also raised serious conceptual issues in interpreting these studies as reflecting consciousness (Blake, Brascamp, and Heeger 2014).

One problem is that when an image is dominant during rivalry, there are other consequences besides our conscious perception of it. For instance, in some studies of binocular rivalry, researchers asked subjects to detect a small change in the two images (Fox and Check 1968; Wales and Fox 1970; Norman, Norman, and Bilotta 2000). Unsurprisingly, subjects could do the task very well, if the change occurred in the dominant image; when we consciously see an image, detecting a small change in it should be easy. However, when the image was in suppression, subjects could also do the detection task above chance. That is, even though the subjects were consciously seeing the dominant image, they could nonetheless detect the small change in the suppressed image. Naturally, this performance was poorer than the performance for the dominant image. So we can think of this as a *performance-capacity confounder*. That is, for an image in dominance, we not only consciously see it but also are able to perform tasks better regarding the image content.

This confounder of performance capacity is important, and yet far from straightforward. In fact, some may think this is not a confounder at all. For example, one may argue that the confounder is only there when we ask subjects to detect the small change. There is no such task in typical binocular rivalry experiments and, therefore, no performance confounder to speak of. But this argument is a bit like saying that we can avoid a confounder by turning a blind eye to it. The emphasis here is on performance *capacity*. Presumably, there is an increased internal perceptual signal strength under perceptual dominance driving this *potential* performance superiority. Even when we don't measure it, the signal difference between dominance and suppression is there, and it could cloud what we may interpret as reflecting subjective experience.

Others may argue that having this superior performance capacity, and a stronger internal perceptual signal, is just a natural consequence of being conscious of the relevant perceptual information. This is what consciousness amounts to. Controlling for such confounders would be like controlling for the length of one's bones as we compare people of different heights; recall our example from Section 1.8 in the Chapter 1.

But there is also a strong disanalogy between these cases. When we compare people with different heights there is simply no way we could control for the length of people's bones. This is because tall people *always* have longer bones. This is what being tall is about. But when it comes to performance capacity, or internal perceptual signal strength, they are not always higher when one is conscious of the relevant perceptual information. We know this from blindsight, in which a lack of conscious experience is nonetheless associated with fairly high performance capacity, sometimes up to above 80% correct in a two-choice discrimination (Weiskrantz 1997). With physically degraded stimuli, which are nonetheless consciously seen, one often performs worse (Persaud et al. 2011). In Section 2.11, we will discuss more examples of how this performance-capacity confounder has been controlled for in actual experiments.

So performance capacity is an important, yet unobvious confounder. In fact, as we will see, it is particularly important *because* it is not obvious.

2.10 Binocular Rivalry as Red Herring

Within the settings of binocular rivalry, it is not so easy to control for performance capacity while assessing subjective experience. But one important study has shed great light on this issue.

Typically in binocular rivalry, we directly ask the subjects to report the percept to assess dominance versus suppression of the images. However, there are indirect methods too. For example, right after an image has been in dominance under rivalry, there are adaptation effects. Adaptation is a well-known phenomenon often exploited in psychophysics (Schwartz, Hsu, and Dayan 2007; Webster 2015). The idea is that after looking at a pattern for some time, an ambiguous stimulus presented at the same location is less likely to look like the pattern. Sometimes we say that the representation for the pattern is *adapted out*. It becomes less likely to win in a perceptual competition, when two alternative percepts are similarly plausible. Therefore, we can indirectly infer which image has been in dominance, based on how a subsequently presented ambiguous stimulus is perceived; it should look less like the image that has been in dominance.

The advantage of using this indirect method of assessing dominance is that we can now test if images rendered invisible may rival too. Zou et al. (2016) used a psychophysical method called flicker fusion to render some images invisible and presented them to the two different eyes. Subjects could not consciously see the images, and, therefore, they could not report what was in dominance or whether there was any rivalry at all. But Zou et al. found that the temporal profile of the adaptation after-effects resembled normal conscious rivalry. An invisible image went into dominance, suppression, and back, in cycles. This must mean that something akin to binocular rivalry happens for the invisible images too. Interestingly, these invisible flicker stimuli activated the visual areas, but not the prefrontal and parietal areas, as measured by their fMRI activity. The prefrontal and parietal areas reacted to the rivalrous stimuli only when they were consciously perceived.

To my mind, these findings from Zou et al. (2016) changed everything regarding the status of binocular rivalry as a tool for studying consciousness (Giles, Lau, and Odegaard 2016). They are very much in favor of the global over the local views. Perhaps these findings are exactly what one would expect, when we consider how the confounder of task performance capacity might have clouded previous results: previous findings of early visual activity reflecting binocular rivalry may just reflect nonconscious rather than conscious signal competitions. These nonconscious signals may compete to drive task performance, but on their own they are not sufficient for consciousness.

2.11 My First Attempt at Taking Down Global Theories

Earlier I mentioned that I am somewhat sympathetic to the global view. But as you will see, this affinity is rather limited. And in fact, it hasn't always been this way.

When I was a young postdoc in London around the mid-2000s, the global view was very much *en vogue*. Being naive and deluded, I took it as my calling to challenge the status quo. In graduate school I understood the point of blindsight, which is that subjective experience and task performance capacity can come apart. So, naturally, I thought we needed to deal with this tricky confounder of performance capacity.

Together with an outstanding undergraduate student, Navindra Persaud, and others, we scanned the blindsight patient GY using fMRI. With a V1 lesion restricted to the left hemisphere, GY was only blindsighted for the right visual field. This means that within the same subject, we can compare blindsight against normal vision (the left visual field). We presented a physically weaker stimulus to the normal, intact hemisphere, and the same stimulus at a higher luminance contrast to the damaged hemisphere. At these psychophysically titrated intensities, GY's performance score on a discrimination task was nearly equal for the two hemifields. And yet, he remained nonconscious of the stimulus in the blind field, while acknowledging that he saw the stimulus consciously about half of the time in the normal field. By comparing stimulation to the different hemispheres, that is, normal vision versus blindsight, we found activations in the prefrontal and parietal cortices, as they are typically found in studies of conscious perception. What was novel though, is that here there was no confounder of task performance capacity, as they were matched between the conditions (Persaud et al. 2011).

Of course, that was from a single patient. But we could do something conceptually similar in subjects from the general population too. Using another "trick" from psychophysics called metacontrast masking, we created conditions under which the subjects' performance in a simple discrimination task was matched. And yet, the target stimuli looked subtly different, as the timing of the masks differed. In one condition, subjects reported that they saw the targets more often than they did in the other condition. Again, comparing the two conditions as we recorded neural activity from the fMRI scanner, we found higher activity in the lateral prefrontal cortex in the condition where subjects said they consciously saw the targets more often (Lau and Passingham 2006).

These findings were somewhat surprising. When I set out to control for performance capacity, I was hoping to challenge the global view. I thought that much of the prefrontal and parietal activations could just reflect one's ability to do the tasks well. In particular, in the metacontrast masking study (Lau and Passingham 2006), the difference in subjective experience was subtle. Subjects only reported seeing the targets consciously about 10% more often in one condition over the other. Despite the fact that it was a visual manipulation (change of mask timing) leading to a visual difference, we couldn't find any activity difference in the visual cortex. This is not to say there was decidedly no difference. With fMRI there is always the issue of sensitivity. Using more invasive methods, I believe we could probably find some differences within the visual cortex too. But it is intriguing that with the limited sensitivity of fMRI, we found an activation in the lateral prefrontal cortex, but not in other areas.

2.12 Why So Hung Up About Performance-Capacity Confounders?

In many ways, the studies described in Section 2.11 are deeply flawed. When we matched for performance capacity, the physical stimulus was no longer matched (Lau and Passingham 2006). To directly control for both performance-capacity and stimulus confounders in the same experiments, one can make use of the phenomenon known as attentional blink. When subjects are asked to detect targets in a rapidly presented series of stimuli, perception is impaired shortly after the detection of a target, as if the subjects need some time to recover. Therefore, when two targets are presented close to each other in time, perception for the second target suffers. Interestingly, this effect seems to be stronger on subjective reports of perception, rather than task-performance capacity itself (Pincham, Bowman, and Szucs 2016; Recht, Mamassian, and de Gardelle 2019). So, like in the study by Lau and Passingham (2006), this provides an opportunity for us to dissociate the two.

Using this task paradigm, Pincham et al. (2016) have measured electrophysical activity on the scalp, and looked at event-related potentials (ERP), a simple and conventional method for analyzing electroencephalogram (EEG) data. In particular, they looked at the ERP time locked to the second target, the visibility of which changed as a function of the temporal distance from the first target, while the physical stimulus itself (for the second target) remained the same. They found that the late-stage ERP component

known as P3 reflected subjective visibility better than objective task performance. This is broadly consistent with the claim that subjective visibility
is associated with downstream processing beyond the sensory cortices. But
as we will see in Section 2.13, this P3 component may be explained by other
confounders.

In the case of blindsight patient GY, we were not only comparing conscious
versus nonconscious vision. We were also comparing an intact versus a damaged hemisphere, and that was admittedly a huge confounder too (Persaud
et al. 2011).

As such, overall, one could rightfully accuse us of merely replacing one set
of confounders (task performance capacity) with several others. But turns
out, this may not be such a bad thing.

This may sound counterintuitive but having an obvious confounder in one's
study is not necessarily so problematic. It may be bad for the individual researcher trying to publish the work. But as a field, we look for converging evidence. Take the case of the stimulus confounder in studies showing that the
prefrontal and parietal areas may be involved in conscious perception. For
example, Dehaene et al.'s study using visually masked words (2001). It is true
that the stimuli were not perfectly matched. But because the confounder was
relatively obvious, other studies have dealt with this problem by presenting a
constant stimulus at around threshold, as well as binocular rivalry. The converging evidence is that the activations in the prefrontal and parietal cortices
under these conditions hold true. As such, these activations are unlikely to be
due to the stimulus confounder alone. Otherwise, studies controlling for the
confounder wouldn't have shown the same results. Therefore, this stimulus
confounder can be considered less fatal to Dehaene et al.'s study. The main
conclusion holds after all.

Contrast this with confounders that are so inconspicuous that the absolute majority of studies in the field do not recognize the need to control for
them. The converging trends from all of these studies could well be commonly
driven by these confounders, and we would be none the wiser. So the main
conclusions, *apparently* replicated over and over, could be at risk.

I worry that performance capacity is exactly one such confounder.
Among hundreds if not thousands of studies on the NCC, I only know of
a few which took the trouble to look into that at all. There is a real danger
there. So it is particularly informative that when the task performance capacity confounder was controlled for, the results were clearly in favor of the
global over the local view.

This may sound like a funny way to defend one's own flawed studies. They
are definitely imperfect, and I don't argue otherwise. But perhaps one could

take this as an argument in favor of diversity in thinking within a field; it may be good that different people worry about different confounders and experimental issues, and we see how the evidence converges overall. As we will see in Chapter 3, these studies matching performance capacity did end up leading to new ideas and findings that together form a coherent story. (Otherwise, I would not be discussing them here, would I?)

2.13 Reports?

The above consideration is also relevant for one recent trend in the literature. So in many of the experiments discussed in the chapter, the subjects were required to make a report, either about the stimulus, or about the experience itself. In everyday life, we don't need to do that. So the task of reporting can be considered a confounder too. Specifically, some of the activity in the prefrontal and parietal cortices may be partially accounted for by this reporting demand, rather than reflecting subjective experience per se (Tsuchiya et al. 2015).

While this is certainly a confounder worth controlling for, the trouble is this is sometimes taken as a "new standard," with the "no-report paradigm" becoming a buzz phrase of some sort. But of course, the recognition of this confounder is nothing new. It has been controlled for in neuroimaging studies of the NCC as early as over 2 decades ago (Lumer and Rees 1999). The typical method is to remove the need for reporting and infer subjective experience in some other indirect ways. Alternatively, one asks the subjects to report on a different stimulus, or a different feature of the stimulus, which is irrelevant to the comparison in questions (e.g., Tse et al. 2005; Mante et al. 2013). In one of such studies using binocular rivalry without report, it was shown that prefrontal and parietal fMRI activations survived such controls (Lumer and Rees 1999). And recent studies using methods with higher sensitivity have repeatedly confirmed this finding in both humans (Vidal et al. 2014; Noy et al. 2015; Huth et al. 2016; Taschereau-Dumouchel, Kawato, and Lau 2019) and monkeys (Panagiotaropoulos et al. 2012; Mante et al. 2013; Panagiotaropoulos, Dwarakanath, and Kapoor 2020).

When reports were not required, there are null findings for prefrontal and parietal activations too (Tse et al. 2005; Kouider et al. 2007; Frässle et al. 2014). But in the light of numerous positive findings, individual negative findings need to be interpreted with care. As a matter of basic statistical consideration, the absence of evidence is not evidence of evidence. Especially with traditional mass-univariate fMRI, sensitivity is limited. It is "easy" to obtain a falsely negative result. Therefore, it would be problematic to claim that these activations are due to nothing but reporting, based on individual null findings. It is particularly troubling when this is presented as if it is a novel, trend-setting discovery.

As we have seen in most of the studies discussed in this chapter, it is probably impossible to have all of the confounders controlled for at once within a single experiment (Michel and Morales 2019). Such a "perfect" experiment probably doesn't exist. In particular, it is not clear how one can control for both the stimulus and performance-capacity confounders under the same conditions. Adding in the reporting confounder makes things more challenging still. As such, fixation on a single confounder is unhelpful. When a certain confounder is considered dealt with, it may be strategically more advantageous to move on and address other confounders. This way, as a field, we can provide more meaningful converging answers.

Having said that, I do think some lessons can be learned from this recent focus on controlling for reports. Earlier I cited studies using invasive neuronal recordings (Panagiotaropoulos et al. 2012; Mante et al. 2013; Panagiotaropoulos, Dwarakanath, and Kapoor 2020). From those studies, it seems like the findings from the prefrontal cortex have survived the control for reports without problem. For other invasive recordings (that are not directly neuronal, but concern local field potentials and related signals), the findings too seem to hold up. However, when reports weren't required, the effect size was significantly reduced (Noy et al. 2015). For fMRI, the story seems similar (Huth et al. 2016). With reduced effect size, occasional null results are exactly as expected.

Earlier I mentioned that the P3 component of the ERP may survive the control of both stimulus and task performance-capacity confounders (Pincham, Bowman, and Szucs 2016). But unfortunately, P3 seems to no longer be present after controlling for task relevance and reporting (Cohen et al. 2020). But once again, this may in part depend on data analysis methods. Using multivariate "decoding" approaches on EEG data, rather than ERP, others have found late-stage correlates, likely reflecting prefrontal activity, which survived similar controls (Sergent et al. 2021).

So the negative findings reviewed here do not falsify the global view. They seem all easily explained by the limited sensitivity of some specific methods. With sufficient sensitivity numerous positive findings were reported. However, it does raise the question of whether the activity in the prefrontal and parietal areas during conscious perception is as widespread and strong as previously thought. If such activity is subtle, the notion that it supports "global ignition" and "broadcast" may seem less plausible (Noy et al. 2015).

2.14. Saying No to No-Cognition

Regarding confounders, Ned Block (2019) has recently suggested we take things one step further: We should employ what he calls "no-cognition paradigms," to rule out that our findings on the NCC may just be due to postperceptual cognitive processes.

The basic rationale seems attractive. It is true that when we consciously see something we tend to think about it, remember it, and contemplate relevant thoughts. Some of these processes are not constitutively part of the subjective experience itself. So it would be good to control for them. But as we see in the last section, when formulated as a general prescription, this kind of "no-XYZ" paradigms could end up doing more harm than good.

If the issue is about postperceptual cognitive processes, this confounder has already been dealt with in some studies. In one study (Mante et al. 2013), the monkeys had to focus on one feature of a stimulus (color or motion direction of some moving dots, depending on the experimental block), and ignore the other feature. The task was difficult, with some stimuli that were rather ambiguous. So actively thinking about the irrelevant feature would be disadvantageous, and the behavior data confirmed that such cognitive interference from the irrelevant feature was in fact small. This was conducted while the researchers recorded signals directly from many neurons in the prefrontal cortex. They found that the neuronal activity reflected the task irrelevant feature—almost as well as it did for the task relevant feature. Even if the monkey did think about the irrelevant feature now and then, the cognitive processes involved were unlikely to be so consistently strong to account for the findings.

In other studies, the monkeys did not have to perform any overt task. They just passively viewed a binocular rivalry display, where perceptual dominance was inferred indirectly. Again, prefrontal activity clearly tracked the dominant percept. Block (2020) argued that perhaps post–perceptual cognition could explain the findings: although the monkeys were not required to think about the percept, they might be "bored" and did so anyway. But as Fanis Panagiotaropoulos and colleagues (2020) pointed out, if the monkeys engaged in such thinking out of boredom, one should expect this to occur somewhat randomly, as wandering thoughts are. But the electrophysiological findings were highly consistent over trials.

Also, prefrontal activity during binocular rivalry often occurs prior to the switch (Dwarakanath et al. 2020). Others have shown that disrupting prefrontal activity causally influences perceptual rivalry as well (Vernet et al.

2015). So, such activity is unlikely to reflect cognition in *reaction* to the perceptual switch. Instead, it seems to be part of the causal process (Weilnhammer et al. 2021).

So we can rule out that the findings were merely due to the animals' explicitly thinking about the percept, in ways that are not constitutively part of the subjective experience itself (i.e., postperceptual thinking). But if the demand is that we need to rule out *any* kind of cognitive process, as the phrase "no-cognition" may suggest, we have to be careful. Recall from Section 1.6 of Chapter 1: We cannot define *consciousness* as entirely independent from cognitive access from the outset. Subjective experience may turn out to constitutively involve some degree of cognition. We have to give such empirical possibilities a fair chance.

Or perhaps Ned Block's intention was not to explicitly beg the question, by ruling out any form of cognition from the outset. Perhaps his point was that we should focus on perceptual events that the subjects do not explicitly "notice," in order to minimize the contamination from attention. But the question of whether unnoticed or unattended perceptual stimuli contribute to our subjective experience is controversial. We will address this in Chapter 4.

2.15 Chapter Summary

This chapter is about the first of the five issues setting the global and local views apart: the neural substrate for subjective experience. We've covered a lot of ground. Some summary is in order.

The central point here revolves around the theme of experimental confounders. Some confounders are unfortunately more "fashionable" than others. But trends come and go. We have to think about what lasts and what matters. Because focusing on addressing a certain confounder will favor some findings over others, this can impact our theoretical views as well. So these discussions can get sectarian pretty quick. We need to see the futility in fighting over which confounders are more important. All confounders are important, and they all need to be addressed. But because it is difficult to address all of them at once in a single experiment, the best way is to consider them in turn, one after another, to aim for an overall broad picture.

If we focus on stimulus and report confounders alone, the overall findings may appear to be in favor of local views. Early sensory activity seems to reflect subjective experiences, even when these two confounders are controlled for: for example, in experiments using binocular rivalry.

The problem, though, is with the confounder of performance capacity. In an experiment where performance capacity was explicitly matched, early sensory activity no longer reflected the difference in reported subjective experience between conditions. Unfortunately, too few studies have controlled for performance capacity, so this negative finding alone may seem indecisive. But in nonconscious binocular rivalry, the early visual activity seems to behave just as it did in ordinary conscious rivalry (Jiang, Zhou, and He 2007). This means that such activity is not always conscious. It may very well just reflect nonconscious internal perceptual signals supporting performance capacity rather than subjective experience. And then, there are also some cases of visual illusions, in which such early visual activity did not track subjective perception well at all. So in sum, it is difficult to say that early sensory activity alone is the NCC.

The global view also does fine regarding the stimulus confound. Many binocular rivalry and near-threshold presentation experiments support the role of prefrontal and parietal activity in subjective perception. Compared to the local view, it fares considerably better with respect to the confounder of task-performance capacity. Admittedly the view also faces considerable challenges with the confounder of reports. But some activity, in particular in the lateral prefrontal cortex, survives such controls—even if such activity may be more subtle and less widespread than previously thought.

These neuroimaging and invasive electrophysiological studies give a rather different picture from what one may intuit based on lesion studies alone. The classical neurological phenomenon of blindsight is associated with damage to V1. However, lesions can have distal effects. We have also gone through the conceptual issues involved in the very definition of the NCC. The main lesson is that considering lesion studies in isolation can be misleading. Accordingly, Larry Weiskrantz, who coined the term *blindsight*, also argued that the mechanisms for subjective visual awareness may well reside within the prefrontal cortex rather than V1 (1997).

In Chapter 3 we will discuss more about lesions and focus on damages to the prefrontal cortex in particular.

References

Bhandari A, Gagne C, Badre D. Just above chance: Is it harder to decode information from prefrontal cortex hemodynamic activity patterns? *J Cogn Neurosci* 2018;**30**:1473–1498.

Binetti N, Tomassini A, Friston K et al. Uncoupling sensation and perception in human time processing. *J Cogn Neurosci* 2020;**32**:1369–1380.

Blake R, Brascamp J, Heeger DJ. Can binocular rivalry reveal neural correlates of consciousness? *Philos Trans R Soc Lond B Biol Sci* 2014;**369**:20130211.

Block N. What is wrong with the no-report paradigm and how to fix it. *Trends Cogn Sci* 2019;**23**:1003–1013.

Block N. Finessing the bored monkey problem. *Trends Cogn Sci* 2020;**24**:167–168.

Boyer JL, Harrison S, Ro T. Unconscious processing of orientation and color without primary visual cortex. *Proc Natl Acad Sci U S A* 2005;**102**:16875–16879.

Bridge H, Harrold S, Holmes EA et al. Vivid visual mental imagery in the absence of the primary visual cortex. *J Neurol* 2012;**259**:1062–1070.

Carmel D, Lavie N, Rees G. Conscious awareness of flicker in humans involves frontal and parietal cortex. *Curr Biol* 2006;**16**:907–911.

Chalmers DJ. What is a neural correlate of consciousness? In: Metzinger T (ed.). *Neural Correlates of Consciousness: Empirical and Conceptual Questions*. MIT Press, 2000.

Cohen MA, Ortego K, Kyroudis A et al. Distinguishing the neural correlates of perceptual awareness and postperceptual processing. *J Neurosci* 2020;**40**:4925–4935.

Craver CF. *Explaining the Brain: Mechanisms and the Mosaic Unity of Neuroscience*. Oxford University Press, 2007.

Dehaene S. *Consciousness and the Brain: Deciphering How the Brain Codes Our Thoughts*. Penguin, 2014.

Dehaene S, Lau H, Kouider S. What is consciousness, and could machines have it? *Science* 2017;**358**:486–492.

Dehaene S, Naccache L, Cohen L et al. Cerebral mechanisms of word masking and unconscious repetition priming. *Nat Neurosci* 2001;**4**:752–758.

Dwarakanath A, Kapoor V, Werner J et al. Prefrontal state fluctuations control access to consciousness. *bioRxiv* 2020.01.29.924928. https://doi.org/10.1101/2020.01.29.924928.

Eagleman DM, Jacobson JE, Sejnowski TJ. Perceived luminance depends on temporal context. *Nature* 2004;**428**:854–856.

Fisch L, Privman E, Ramot M et al. Neural "ignition": Enhanced activation linked to perceptual awareness in human ventral stream visual cortex. *Neuron* 2009;**64**:562–574.

Fox R, Check R. Detection of motion during binocular rivalry suppression. *J Exp Psychol* 1968;**78**:388–395.

Frässle S, Sommer J, Jansen A et al. Binocular rivalry: frontal activity relates to introspection and action but not to perception. *J Neurosci* 2014;**34**:1738–1747.

Giles N, Lau H, Odegaard B. What type of awareness does binocular rivalry assess? *Trends Cogn Sci* 2016;**20**:719–720.

Gotts SJ, Chow CC, Martin A. Repetition priming and repetition suppression: A case for enhanced efficiency through neural synchronization. *Cogn Neurosci* 2012;**3**:227–237.

Huang L, Wang L, Shen W et al. A source for awareness-dependent figure-ground segregation in human prefrontal cortex. *Proc Natl Acad Sci U S A* 2020;**117**:30836–30847.

Huth AG, Lee T, Nishimoto S et al. Decoding the semantic content of natural movies from human brain activity. *Front Syst Neurosci* 2016;**10**:81.

Jiang Y, Zhou K, He S. Human visual cortex responds to invisible chromatic flicker. *Nat Neurosci* 2007;**10**:657–662.

Kouider S, Dehaene S, Jobert A et al. Cerebral bases of subliminal and supraliminal priming during reading. *Cereb Cortex* 2007;**17**:2019–2029.

Lamme VA. Blindsight: The role of feedforward and feedback corticocortical connections. *Acta Psychol* 2001;**107**:209–228.

Lamme VAF. Why visual attention and awareness are different. *Trends Cogn Sci* 2003;**7**:12–18.

Lau HC, Brown R. The emperor's new phenomenology? The empirical case for conscious experiences without first-order representations. In A Pautz and D Stoljar (Eds), Blockheads! MIT Press, 2019, Chapter 11.

Lau HC, Passingham RE. Relative blindsight in normal observers and the neural correlate of visual consciousness. *Proc Natl Acad Sci U S A* 2006;**103**:18763–18768.

LeDoux JE, Michel M, Lau H. A little history goes a long way toward understanding why we study consciousness the way we do today. *Proc Natl Acad Sci U S A* 2020;**117**:6976–6984.

Liu S, Yu Q, Tse PU et al. Neural correlates of the conscious perception of visual location lie outside visual cortex. *Curr Biol* 2019;**29**:4036–4044.e4.

Lumer ED, Rees G. Covariation of activity in visual and prefrontal cortex associated with subjective visual perception. *Proc Natl Acad Sci U S A* 1999;**96**:1669–1673.

Macknik SL, Martinez-Conde S. The role of feedback in visual masking and visual processing. *Adv Cogn Psychol* 2008;**3**:125–52.

Malach R. Conscious perception and the frontal lobes: Comment on Lau and Rosenthal. *Trends Cogn Sci* 2011;**15**:507; author reply 508–9.

Mante V, Sussillo D, Shenoy KV et al. Context-dependent computation by recurrent dynamics in prefrontal cortex. *Nature* 2013;**503**:78–84.

Mazzi C, Savazzi S, Silvanto J. On the "blindness" of blindsight: What is the evidence for phenomenal awareness in the absence of primary visual cortex (V1)? *Neuropsychologia* 2019;**128**:103–108.

Michel M. Consciousness science underdetermined: A short history of endless debates. *Ergo* 2019;**6**. https://doi.org/10.3998/ergo.12405314.0006.028.

Michel M, Doerig A. A new empirical challenge for local theories of consciousness. *Mind Lang* 2021. https://doi.org/10.1111/mila.12319.

Michel M, Lau H. On the dangers of conflating strong and weak versions of a theory of consciousness. *PhiMiSci* 2020. https://doi.org/ 0.33735/phimisci.2020.II.54.

Michel M, Morales J. Minority reports: Consciousness and the prefrontal cortex. *Mind Lang* 2019, https://doi.org/10.1111/mila.12264.

Miller SM. Closing in on the constitution of consciousness. *Front Psychol* 2014;5:1293.

Norman HF, Norman JF, Bilotta J. The temporal course of suppression during binocular rivalry. *Perception* 2000;29:831–841.

Noy N, Bickel S, Zion-Golumbic E et al. Ignition's glow: Ultra-fast spread of global cortical activity accompanying local "ignitions" in visual cortex during conscious visual perception. *Conscious Cogn* 2015;**35**:206–224.

Odegaard B, Knight RT, Lau H. Should a few null findings falsify prefrontal theories of conscious perception? *J Neurosci* 2017;**37**:9593–9602.

Panagiotaropoulos TI, Deco G, Kapoor V et al. Neuronal discharges and gamma oscillations explicitly reflect visual consciousness in the lateral prefrontal cortex. *Neuron* 2012;**74**:924–935.

Panagiotaropoulos TI, Dwarakanath A, Kapoor V. Prefrontal cortex and consciousness: Beware of the signals. *Trends Cogn Sci* 2020;**24**:343–344.

Pascual-Leone A, Walsh V. Fast backprojections from the motion to the primary visual area necessary for visual awareness. *Science* 2001;**292**:510–512.

Persaud N, Davidson M, Maniscalco B et al. Awareness-related activity in prefrontal and parietal cortices in blindsight reflects more than superior visual performance. *Neuroimage* 2011;**58**:605–611.

Pincham HL, Bowman H, Szucs D. The experiential blink: Mapping the cost of working memory encoding onto conscious perception in the attentional blink. *Cortex* 2016;**81**:35–49.

Place UT. Is consciousness a brain process? *Br J Psychol* 1956:47: 44–50.

Recht S, Mamassian P, de Gardelle V. Temporal attention causes systematic biases in visual confidence. *Sci Rep* 2019;**9**:11622.

Rees G, Kreiman G, Koch C. Neural correlates of consciousness in humans. *Nat Rev Neurosci* 2002;**3**:261–270.

Ro T, Harrison S, Boyer J et al. Unconscious orientation and color processing without primary visual cortex. *J Vis* 2010;5:285–285.

Sandberg K, Bahrami B, Kanai R et al. Early visual responses predict conscious face perception within and between subjects during binocular rivalry. *J Cogn Neurosci* 2013;**25**:969–985.

Schwartz O, Hsu A, Dayan P. Space and time in visual context. *Nat Rev Neurosci* 2007;**8**:522–535.

Schwarzkopf DS, Schindler A, Rees G. Knowing with which eye we see: Utrocular discrimination and eye-specific signals in human visual cortex. *PLOS One* 2010;5:e13775.

Sergent C, Corazzol M, Labouret G et al. Bifurcation in brain dynamics reveals a signature of conscious processing independent of report. *Nat Commun* 2021;12:1149.

Silvanto J. Why is "blindsight" blind? A new perspective on primary visual cortex, recurrent activity and visual awareness. *Conscious Cogn* 2015;32:15–32.

Taschereau-Dumouchel V, Kawato M, Lau H. Multivoxel pattern analysis reveals dissociations between subjective fear and its physiological correlates. *Mol Psychiatry* 2019. https://doi.org/10.1038/s41380-019-0520-3.

Tong F. Primary visual cortex and visual awareness. *Nat Rev Neurosci* 2003;4:219–229.

Tse PU, Martinez-Conde S, Schlegel AA et al. Visibility, visual awareness, and visual masking of simple unattended targets are confined to areas in the occipital cortex beyond human V1/V2. *Proc Natl Acad Sci U S A* 2005;102:17178–17183.

Tsuchiya N, Wilke M, Frässle S et al. No-Report Paradigms: Extracting the True Neural Correlates of Consciousness. *Trends Cogn Sci* 2015;19:757–770.

Vernet M, Brem A-K, Farzan F et al. Synchronous and opposite roles of the parietal and prefrontal cortices in bistable perception: A double-coil TMS-EEG study. *Cortex* 2015;64:78–88.

Vidal JR, Perrone-Bertolotti M, Kahane P et al. Intracranial spectral amplitude dynamics of perceptual suppression in fronto-insular, occipito-temporal, and primary visual cortex. *Front Psychol* 2014;5:1545.

Wales R, Fox R. Increment detection thresholds during binocular rivalry suppression. *Percept Psychophys* 1970;8:90–94.

Webster MA. Visual Adaptation. *Annu Rev Vis Sci* 2015;1:547–567.

Weilnhammer V, Fritsch M, Chikermane M et al. An active role of inferior frontal cortex in conscious experience. *Curr Biol* 2021;31:2868–2880.e8.

Weiskrantz L. *Consciousness Lost and Found.* Oxford University Press, 1997.

Zhang X, Zhaoping L, Zhou T et al. Neural activities in v1 create a bottom-up saliency map. *Neuron* 2012;73:183–192.

Zhou H, Davidson M, Kok P et al. Spatiotemporal dynamics of brightness coding in human visual cortex revealed by the temporal context effect. *Neuroimage* 2020;205:116277.

Zou J, He S, Zhang P. Binocular rivalry from invisible patterns. *Proc Natl Acad Sci U S A* 2016;113:8408–8013.

3

Hitting the Right Note

3.1 Prefrontal Cortex Versus the Rest of the Brain

Why the prefrontal cortex may be particularly important for subjective perceptual experiences was outlined in Chapter 2. In particular, the concerned areas include the dorsolateral prefrontal areas and the frontal polar cortex (Figure 3.1). These regions are identified as important because they seem to have survived the controls for all three kinds of confounders discussed in this volume: stimulus, report, and performance.

However, there have been relatively few studies controlling for the confounders of task-performance capacity. So we have to keep this caveat in mind. Perhaps future studies using methods that are more sensitive may reveal that some other areas, possibly outside of the prefrontal cortex, may survive the control of this confounder too.

At the theoretical level, it is worth emphasizing that global theories do not fixate on these prefrontal areas alone. Other prefrontal regions, such as the anterior cingulate, have also been included in previous discussion (Dehaene 2014; Mashour et al. 2020). Specific parietal areas are densely connected to their lateral prefrontal "counterparts," so, functionally, they often work together (Katsuki 2012). As such, these areas are likely relevant too, according to global theories. So the divide between local and global, really concerns early sensory regions, versus later areas in the association cortex (including both the prefrontal and parietal areas).

Having said that, the prefrontal cortex is often a key focus in current debates. One of the main reasons is that some authors have made strong statements on its exclusion from the neural correlates of consciousness (NCC) (Koch et al. 2016). For example, it has been suggested that the entire frontal lobes, together with the insular, hippocampus, amygdala, and claustrumc—that is, all the areas in the anterior portion of the entire brain—are all not constitutively involved in *any* kind of subjective experience, and not just visual experiences (Koch 2018). Presumably, this includes emotions, sense of volition, conscious recollection of past memories, hunger, interoception, and bodily arousal, for example. This may seem surprising in the light of current

In Consciousness We Trust. Hakwan Lau, Oxford University Press. © Hakwan Lau 2022.
DOI: 10.1093/oso/9780198856771.003.0004

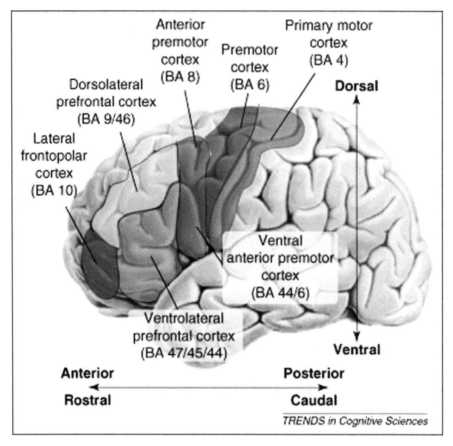

Figure 3.1   Different subregions within the prefrontal cortex

standard textbook knowledge (Gazzaniga 2009; Kandel 2013). These same authors are also not so clear about exactly where the NCC may be. At times they invoke phrases such as *posterior hot zone* or *posterior cortex*. But these are neither standard nor specific anatomical labels. So, in the context of visual awareness, their main agenda seems to be just to rule out other anterior areas. Given the evidence reviewed in Chapter 2, these claims may be puzzling. Here we discuss how such confusion might have come about.

3.2   Conceptual Confusions About Lesions

One main argument against the prefrontal cortex as part of the NCC has to do with lesion effects (Pollen 2008; Koch et al. 2016). Damage to the prefrontal cortex does not lead to functional blindness nor total loss of sense of smell, taste, touch, and so on. So the prefrontal cortex can't be critically important for subjective experiences, the argument goes.

But how do we account for the activity found in the prefrontal cortex in neuroimaging and invasive recording studies on conscious perception? Interestingly, the authors who make the lesion argument often say that such activity may be due to the reporting confounder (Koch et al. 2016). That is, the activity may be driven by the fact that subjects had to report about what they saw, rather than conscious experience per se. But there seems to be a logical contradiction, as pointed out by Michel and Morales (2019): if the prefrontal activity reflected report rather than subjective experience, shouldn't damages to the area abolish the subjects' ability to make these reports? If so, wouldn't these subjects perform poorly in perceptual tasks, as they fail to make reports? And yet, this is typically not what was found in these patients. As pointed out by these same authors (Koch et al. 2016), the patients can do these tasks very well.

The way to resolve this contradiction is to recognize: lesions do not always abolish the relevant mechanisms causally supported by the region (Jonas and Kording 2017). We have already mentioned this point in Section 2.3 of Chapter 2. This really is standard knowledge not only in cognitive neuroscience, but biology in general. In particular, the notion of degeneracy refers to the fact that in biological systems, multiple parallel mechanisms can support a similar function (Mason 2010). These mechanisms are unlikely to be exactly identical in every aspect, so strictly speaking, this is not to say evolution has given us straight-up redundancy. But all the same, within the context of a specific function, these mechanisms are close enough that they can often serve as "backup" for one another, at least to some extent. So knocking out a substrate for one mechanism may not completely abolish the function. The lack of abolishment of function does not mean that the substrate is causally irrelevant.

Specifically, we expect the level of degeneracy to be high for systems of high complexity, as defined by how different units are connected to each other (Tononi, Sporns, and Edelman 1999). The dorsolateral prefrontal areas are widely connected to many other regions (Petrides and Pandya 2002), and some of their connected areas, such as those in the parietal cortex that, in turn, have rather similar connectivity profiles (i.e., the pattern of connections with respect to all other areas) (Katsuki 2012). So these areas are in a sense central in the entire network, and yet they aren't uniquely irreplaceable. When we look at such a "circuit diagram," we should already expect these areas to show higher levels of degeneracy than others. Recent neuroimaging work has exploited this insight, to predict the severity of lesion effects based on the connectivity profile of the damaged brain region in the network (Alstott et al. 2009; Lim, Hutchings, and Kaiser 2017).

Theoretical expectations aside, studies have also *empirically* demonstrated that after a unilateral lesion to the prefrontal cortex, areas in the opposite hemisphere can dynamically change their activity to compensate for the effect of the lesion (Voytek et al. 2010).

This is of course not to say all prefrontal functions show this kind of resistance to structural damage. One of the most established neuropsychological findings is that damage to specific areas in the left ventral prefrontal cortex (the so-called Broca's area) can completely abolish language production (Musso et al. 2003). But such highly lateralized function is the exception rather than the rule, as far as the prefrontal cortex is concerned. The exceptional nature of such lesion effects is also predicted by the pattern of anatomical connectivity in the concerned language areas, with the same rationale described earlier.

So we should not expect unilateral lesions to prefrontal areas implicated in previous NCC studies to lead to dramatic "knockout" effects, either on report or subjective experience. For these areas (dorsolateral and frontal pole), the anatomical connections and functions are less lateralized (Croxson et al. 2005). Unlike in language, when one side is damaged, the other may serve as "backup," at least to some extent.

3.3 Controversial Case Studies

But how about bilateral lesions? After such lesions, perhaps there is still the possibility that the connected parietal areas can take over as backup. In monkeys, it has been shown that when both the relevant prefrontal and parietal areas were damaged, the animals indeed behaved functionally blind (Nakamura and Mishkin 1986). In fact, such lesions do not need to be bilateral. Unilateral damage to the left hemisphere, together with damage to the optic tract and the corpus callosum, which prevented visual information from going through the other hemisphere, were sufficient to render the animals functionally blind.

In humans, of course, such carefully planned lesions cannot be performed for experimental purposes. But one may expect that if naturally occurring prefrontal lesions (e.g., because of stroke or external trauma) are bilateral and large, the extent to which the parietal cortices can fully compensate for their functions should be somewhat limited. If the global view is right, we should at least expect some noticeable effect of such large bilateral lesions on subjective experience.

Unfortunately, many false claims have been made in the literature concerning these patient cases. Turns out, in most cases, the lesions were incomplete. The most critical areas concerned here (e.g., dorsolateral pre-frontal cortex) were often spared (Odegaard, Knight, and Lau 2017). In a much discussed case (Patient A), it was reported that the patient behaved just as normal, even after complete bilateral removal of the entire frontal lobes (Boly et al. 2017). But the alleged normal behavior is not consistent with other details reported. Rather, "when anything but the most casual attention is dir-ected upon [the patient], peculiarities in his behavior rapidly become mani-fest" (Brickner 1936).

More importantly, as the figure from the original report clearly shows, large parts of the prefrontal cortex actually remained intact postmortem (Brickner 1952). So the intended surgical lesion, performed back in the days before the guidance of neuroimaging, was likely inadvertently incomplete. The doctor also referred to the lobectomy as "partial" rather than "complete" (subtitle of Brickner's 1936 book about the patient case). And yet, inaccurate versions of these "stories," sometimes involving anatomical claims grossly incompatible with textbook knowledge, continue to be told through secondary sources in the literature.

For a more in-depth review of these controversies, the readers can see Odegaard et al. (2017), including our reply to Boly et al. (2017) in that ex-change. In our paper, there is also a link to the video of a patient with truly complete bilateral lesions to the lateral prefrontal areas, as confirmed by modern magnetic resonance imaging. The video showed the patient's behavior as he was tested by our coauthor Bob Knight. It is evident that the patient was largely unresponsive. To the extent that there were some simple reactions to verbal commands, it is difficult to ascertain if they were mere reflexes. This is not to say we can establish that the patient lacked subjective experiences en-tirely, or even partially. But the point is exactly that: addressing this question empirically in such cases is extremely difficult.

3.4 Choosing the Right Behavioral Measure

So single patient cases can be controversial. Of course, this is true even in some "classic" and well-documented cases, for example, in studies of amnesia. Often, details are revisited, leading to new interpretations (Stanley and Krakauer 2013; De Brigard 2019). Therefore, it is useful to study the phenomena in a larger cohort of subjects, ideally in settings that are more controlled.

Having tried and failed to find enough suitable patients to be tested, in the mid-2000s, I set out to address the question with a different method: transcranial magnetic stimulation (TMS). Using TMS, under the right setup, we can try to create so-called "virtual lesions" (i.e., temporary suppression of the neural activity in a brain area). This way we can experimentally induce causal interventions in subjects from the general population.

However, as I was planning the study, several senior colleagues warned me that it probably wouldn't work. I appreciated the advice because they were kindly sharing their own experiences with me. The message was that they had tried, and it just didn't work.

I still believe what they said was true. But my question was: *what* didn't work? With TMS to the prefrontal cortex, we don't expect dramatic effects such as complete abolishment of visual functions. Prefrontal functions are not specific to a sensory modality. If the effects are so strong as to completely abolish the functions, even temporarily, perhaps nobody should participate in these studies! As such, at a level of intensity where the stimulation is safe, we just can't expect the subjects to spontaneously tell us something changed drastically. The effects are unlikely to be so big.

More importantly, if we follow the logic of the experiments described in Chapter 2 (Section 2.11), perhaps what one should expect is not that TMS to the prefrontal cortex would impair visual task performance. Rather, the idea is that it may selectively impair self-reports of subjective experience. That is, subjects may say they see the visual targets less clearly, or maybe they are merely guessing on some trials—while their ability to press keys to correctly discriminate the stimulus may not change much, if at all.

Turns out, visual task performance was indeed what my colleagues had focused on in their earlier attempts. This may sound surprising in this context, but in vision science, we tend to focus on task-performance capacity—not as a confounder, but as the measurement of interest. Sometimes we even go out of our way to use analytic tools such as signal detection theory to *remove* the influence of subjective "biases" to focus on "uncontaminated" effects of performance capacity (Peters, Ro, and Lau 2016). The origin of this tradition is complex, in part because of the different purposes of common experiments. There are also historical reasons. But in any case, since my hope was to find a different kind of effect—of subjective reports of experience rather than discrimination task performance—their warning me that it didn't work in their experiments somehow encouraged me to try it out.

3.5 Stumbled Upon Metacognition

It was my collaborator Elisabeth Rounis who ran the study. Together with John Rothwell and others, their lab pioneered a protocol of stimulation known as "theta-burst." The details aren't important, but after a minute or so of stimulation, they can make a brain area less responsive for up to an hour (Huang et al. 2005). This is handy because usually you don't want to stimulate both sides of the prefrontal cortex simultaneously, for the risk of inducing seizure. But here, one could stimulate one side, wait a bit, and then stimulate the other side. Afterward, we should expect that both sides of the prefrontal cortex become less responsive.

Just as my colleagues expected, TMS did virtually nothing to the visual task performance; the stimulus intensity required for subjects to achieve a near-threshold performance remained the same before and after TMS. However, TMS changed the correlations between the subjective ratings of visibility and performance. In other words, usually after people reported that they saw the stimulus clearly on a trial, they were more likely to be correct in discriminating what the stimulus was. We can say that this across-trials association between subjective ratings and accuracy measures *metacognition*, following the convention in studies of memory and learning (Rhodes and Castel 2009; Metcalfe and Son 2012). Using this measure, metacognition in visual perception was found to be lowered after TMS (Rounis et al. 2010).

But how big was the effect? Given that TMS did little to discrimination task performance, perhaps we shouldn't expect the effect on visual metacognition to be very large. But quantifying the magnitude of this effect was not trivial. Typical correlation measures do not suffice, as they will be influenced by very many factors not of our interest. Fortunately, I had an extraordinarily brilliant research assistant in my laboratory at Columbia University at that time. Using signal detection theory, Brian Maniscalco developed the measure meta-d', now rather commonly used in studies of this sort (Maniscalco and Lau 2012). With this measure, we can precisely assess how far a subject is away from "ideal" metacognitive efficiency. We found that before TMS, people were nearly perfect. After TMS, this metacognitive efficiency dropped by over 20% (Rounis et al. 2010).

A TMS effect of 20% change in a behavioral measure isn't exactly small. Some have found that the direction of this effect seems to depend subtly on the exact location of stimulation; TMS to the frontal polar area, anterior to where Rounis et al. targeted, boosted rather than impaired metacognition in one study (Rahnev et al. 2016). This is consistent with more recent findings that mechanisms for metacognition likely depend on spatially distributed patterns of activity within the lateral prefrontal and parietal areas (Cortese et al. 2016). We should not think of prefrontal activity as representing the "intensity" of metacognition. The prefrontal cortex is complex, and certainly not a simple signaling device. We will come back to this point in Section 3.11.

Others have challenged that this effect may not be replicable (Bor et al. 2017). But turns out, the alleged nonreplicability was observed only after the authors discarded data that they did not consider "good" enough. If they did not discard the data, a significant positive finding was actually found. I think the intention to focus on "good" data should be applauded, but a computational simulation analysis showed that the criteria chosen for discarding such data do not actually improve the authors' ability to reject false positive results (Ruby, Maniscalco, and Peters 2018). Nor does it improve their statistical power, which was low to begin with, in both the original study and the attempted "replication." At low power, even if the effect is real, the chance of missing it is high. So from a statistical point of view, despite the good intention, it's unclear what was the basis of their claims. And a null result would have been difficult to interpret in any case (because of limited statistical power).

Fortunately, the result that disruption of prefrontal activity can lead to impairment of metacognition has now been observed in studies across many labs and species, including lesions in humans (Fleming et al. 2014), and chemical inactivations (via muscimol injections, which lead to temporary disruptions of neuronal activity in the area) in both monkeys (Miyamoto et al. 2017) and rats (Lak et al. 2014). Martijn Wokke (personal communication) likewise replicated the finding using the same TMS protocol (i.e., theta-burst), targeting the same brain region (i.e., dorsolateral prefrontal area) in humans. Another TMS study has reported that stimulation to this region likely lowered subjective confidence in a visual task, leading to more reported "guesses" (Chiang et al. 2014). Also using TMS, Lapate et al. (2019) found that stimulation to this area impaired metacognition in a perceptual judgment (i.e., whether a face was upright or inverted), but not affective judgment (i.e., concerning the emotions expressed by the face). Targeting slightly different prefrontal areas (i.e., more anterior to dorsolateral prefrontal cortex) with TMS, others have also found selective effects on metacognition in perceptual tasks (Rahnev et al. 2016; Miyamoto et al. 2021).

So the finding seems to hold up. But this is not to say my original study was well-conceived. There were admittedly many flaws. As I mentioned, I did it somewhat out of spite, as a young postdoc trying to show that my senior colleagues were wrong. But thanks to my brilliant collaborators, somehow it worked. This theme is to repeat itself very many times: a rather poorly conceived idea of mine, leading to something empirically replicable and insightful somehow, owing to the sheer luck of having great people working with me (Rounis et al. 2010; Maniscalco and Lau 2012).

3.6 More Windfall: Specific Lesion Effects

To be frank, I was initially not so sure about the TMS result. We set out looking for an effect on subjective experience, based on the neuroimaging studies reviewed in Section 3.5. But we ended up finding an effect on perceptual metacognition. Are the two related at all? In the paper, we said TMS changed "metacognitive awareness." But I have come to admit that it was a bit of a stretch.

Meanwhile, Steve Fleming in London has looked at individual differences in gray matter volume in different brain regions, and found that the people with a larger or denser frontal polar cortex were also better at visual metacognition (Fleming et al. 2010). The frontal polar area in question was just slightly anterior to the dorsolateral prefrontal cortex, the region we targeted in our TMS study (Rounis et al. 2010).

I was intrigued by the finding, but assessing individual differences requires large samples. So I was hoping to test if we could replicate these findings. A very outstanding undergraduate student working in my lab, Liyan McCurdy, took up the task. To make it slightly more interesting, we thought we could compare perceptual metacognition with memory metacognition too. As I mentioned earlier, the idea of treating the correlation between confidence and accuracy as a measurement of metacognition came from studies of memory and learning. So we asked people to study a list of words. Later they were given a pair of words, one new, and one from the list they studied. Subjects had to indicate which was which. After that, they rated confidence. We could use the same analysis method (i.e., meta-d') to assess how close they were to metacognitively ideal performance (i.e., how well their confidence ratings maximally distinguished between their correct and incorrect memory responses).

We confirmed Fleming's finding that individual differences in gray matter volume in the frontal polar area reflected visual metacognition (McCurdy et al. 2013). Memory metacognition was instead reflected by variations in gray matter volume in a medial posterior parietal area known as the precuneus. The two behavioral measures correlated weakly. That is, people who were good at visual metacognition tended to be good at memory metacognition too. But that was explained by the fact that people with larger or denser frontal poles also tended to have a larger or denser precuneus (Figure 3.2). Each type of metacognitive behavior (e.g., memory vs perceptual) seems to have their own structural correlates (e.g., precuneus vs frontal pole).

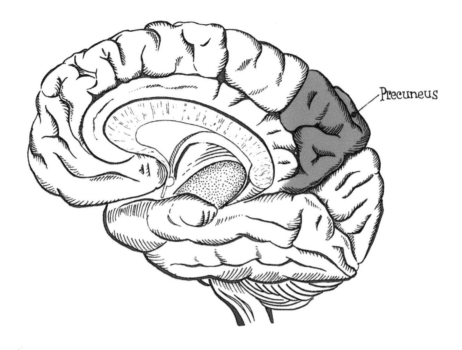

Figure 3.2 A medial parietal region known as the precuenus; besides contributing to memory metacognition, the region seems to also play a role in determining memory vividness (Richter et al. 2016)

Reproduced with permission from Trimble, M. R., and Cavanna, A. E. (2008). The role of the precuneus in episodic memory. *Handbook of Behavioral Neuroscience*, 18, 363-377.

That was all based on statistical analysis, and partly because of that, I confess I did not fully believe the results. One tries to be clean and rigorous about the data collection and analysis, but at the end of the day, I never feel I can trust single studies. The sample size (N = 34) was in line with the standards of the day, but by now we should all recognize its inadequacy. All the same, that's what the data apparently showed. So we wrote up the paper, published it, and hoped to see how it goes (McCurdy et al. 2013).

To my very pleasant surprise, with other colleagues, Steve Fleming later ran a study on patients with unilateral lesions to the prefrontal cortex (2014). Like I mentioned earlier, with unilateral lesions we don't expect very salient effects. But informed by the then recent studies, Steve focused on this same measure of metacognitive efficiency (meta-d') and found that patients with unilateral prefrontal lesions were impaired in visual metacognition by up to about 50%!

To my mind, Fleming et al. (2014) was a landmark study not just because of the magnitude and clarity of the effect. The lesson for me was that perhaps previous patient studies just did not look for the right behavioral measures. More importantly, Steve found that the subjects were virtually unimpaired in a similar memory metacognition task. This confirmed McCurdy et al.'s prediction (2013), that the prefrontal cortex was primarily important for perceptual, but not memory, metacognition. Also, it means that the patients were not just less able to rate confidence, introspect, or the like. The effect was specific to their ability to monitor the effectiveness of their *perceptual* processes. Whatever is impaired, it seems to have something to do with perceptual experiences specifically.

3.7 A Double Dissociation?

McCurdy et al.'s study (2013) didn't just predict the single dissociation, confirmed by Fleming et al.'s lesion study (2014). If the model supported by the statistical analysis was right, we should also expect that lesions to the precuneus would selectively impair perceptual metacognition more than memory metacognition too.

We never got around to testing this with patients with lesions to the precuneus. But with Sze Chai Kwok's lab, we did a study in which we applied TMS targeting to the area. To my pleasant surprise again, it impaired memory but not perceptual metacognition (Ye et al. 2018), just as McCurdy et al. (2013) predicted.

Despite these findings, it would be dishonest of me to claim that we've solidly proven the double dissociation—that prefrontal interruption only impairs perceptual metacognition, and precuneus interruption only impairs memory metacognition. For example, after researchers injected muscimol to the dorsolateral prefrontal cortex in monkeys, which has the effect of temporarily deactivating the area, the animals were impaired in a memory metacognition task (Miyamoto et al. 2017). Again, the basic primary memory performance was relatively unimpaired. So it was specific to metacognition. But based on McCurdy et al.'s model (2013), one would have expected this to affect perceptual metacognition. And yet a memory metacognition effect was found.

Perhaps one interpretation is that the effect was less selective with chemical inactivations. Because the effect was transient, researchers needed to test the animals immediately after. With lesions, the effect is longer lasting. Testing tends not to be carried out immediately following the brain damage. This may be why lesion studies better reveal what functions can or cannot truly recover in the long-term. For all we know, it is possible that right after the lesion, Fleming et al.'s prefrontal patients were impaired in both perceptual and memory metacognition too. But over time, memory metacognition recovered while perceptual metacognition didn't. This interpretation is speculative, of course.

3.8 Parallel Versus Hierarchical Architectures

Regardless of the status of the double dissociation, the prefrontal cortex does seem to be causally involved in perceptual metacognition. But is it trivial? *Metacognition* here refers to the monitoring or self-evaluation of an internal process (e.g., perception or memory). Surely, that is done by some "higher-cognitive" areas in the brain (e.g., the prefrontal cortex)?

The findings are not so trivial in several ways. First we have to emphasize that it was somewhat specific to perceptual but not memory metacognition, at least in some studies (McCurdy et al. 2013; Fleming et al. 2014). So it isn't just about self-monitoring or introspection in general. It has something specifically to do with ongoing perceptual experiences.

Also, in the studies reviewed, metacognition often concerns the simple task of giving meaningful confidence ratings. Others have argued that such representations of confidence can be found within the visual cortex (Ma et al. 2006; van Bergen et al. 2015; Walker et al. 2020). So the role of the prefrontal cortex in these simple "metacognitive" tasks is not uncontested.

In fact, the view that perceptual metacognition requires a higher-order monitoring mechanism is contested even by prominent global theorists. Compare the following two different views: in the first view, we can call the perceptual process supporting one's ability to do basic visual tasks (e.g., discriminate or identify the stimulus itself) a first-order process. Let us postulate a second, later-stage process. We can call this a higher-order process, which may monitor the first-order process, in the sense that this later-stage process receives input from the first-order process. Based on this input, the higher-order process evaluates the quality of the first-order process, and thereby generates the metacognitive response (i.e., confidence). This way we can have a selective change in metacognitive efficiency, while holding basic task performance constant; this is achieved by changing the higher-order process alone. We can call this the hierarchical model. See Figure 3.3, right.

An alternative view is: There may be two *parallel* processes instead. They are not in tandem in a hierarchical structure. They are just somewhat independently working side-by-side. One process may contribute to one's ability to do basic visual tasks without informing our metacognition. We can call this a "nonconscious" process. The other process may contribute to both, which we can call a "conscious" process. This way, we can also have a selective change in metacognitive efficiency, while holding basic task performance constant; this is achieved by changing the balance between the two processes. If the "conscious" process dominates, that is when most of the relevant signals go through it instead of the other process, our metacognition should be well informed. If, on the other hand, most of the signals go through the "nonconscious" process, we can have the same basic task performance overall, but our metacognition may be relatively uninformed. We can call this the parallel model. See Figure 3.3, left.

One of the major proponents of global views, Stan Dehaene, favors the parallel model. This was based on the results from yet another lesion study showing that damages to the prefrontal cortex can impair visual perception (Del Cul et al. 2009). There, unlike in Fleming et al.'s study (2014), basic visual task performance was impaired too. But the impact of prefrontal lesion was more pronounced on the subjective visibility ratings. Dehaene and colleagues wrote out a computational version of the parallel model and fitted it to the patients' behavioral data (see the supplementary materials in Del Cul et al. (2009)). The model accounted for the findings well. The interpretation for these findings is that the "conscious" process is reflected by widespread cortical activities including those in the prefrontal and parietal areas. The "nonconscious" process may be supported by subcortical activities.

In the memory literature, these kinds of parallel models are also popular. In that literature we distinguish between two kinds of memory. When a stimulus remembered from a prior experience is encountered again, we can have conscious episodic recall, where the memory is replayed vividly in our minds.

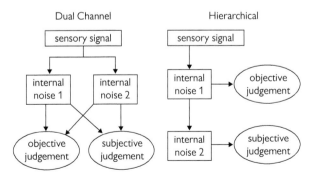

Figure 3.3 Parallel (dual-channel) versus hierarchical models

Reproduced under a Creative Commons Attribution-NonCommercial 4.0 International (CC BY-NC 4.0) from Maniscalco, B. and Lau, H. (2016). The signal processing architecture underlying subjective reports of sensory awareness. *Neurosci Conscious,* 1. https://doi.org/10.1093/nc/niw002

Alternatively, there may merely be an implicit sense of familiarity. To distinguish between the two kinds of memory responses, one often invokes parallel models akin to the model described herein (Yonelinas et al. 2010). The interpretation is that conscious and nonconscious memories depend on distinct neural pathways.

However, just because a model can fit some data does not mean it is the correct model. There may be other models which can provide a better fit of the data while being just as parsimonious (i.e., simple). So we have to directly compare alternative models quantitatively. This is what Brian Maniscalco did. He computationally implemented many variants of the hierarchical and parallel models. He found that the best-fitting model is hierarchical, not parallel (Maniscalco and Lau 2016). We can interpret this as the late-stage higher-order process being reflected by activity in the prefrontal and possibly also parietal cortices. The first-order process may be reflected better by activity in the visual cortex. This is consistent with many results discussed earlier in this chapter, including the TMS, lesion, and inactivation lesions targeting the prefrontal cortex. A change in the higher-order process mainly changes metacognition but not basic task performance itself.

Therefore, perceptual metacognition seems to be supported by a late-stage mechanism. This is neither trivial nor tautological. It was an empirical finding.

3.9 But Is It Really About Consciousness?

As I hinted at earlier, there is a totally fair criticism for what I have discussed so far. The question we started off with in this chapter is whether the prefrontal cortex plays a causal role in conscious perception. But from the discussion of the findings of Rounis et al. (2010), I have gradually shifted my focus toward metacognition. Based on the results of Fleming et al. (2014), I argue that this is specific to perception but not memory. However, it still is perceptual metacognition, not perception itself. What do these findings have to do with subjective experience?

I acknowledge that we should not treat perceptual metacognition as identical to consciousness at all. I presented the studies here as they happened, in part to highlight that the discovery of the empirical connection is somewhat incidental. Sometimes that's the advantage of doing experiments; the data may tell us unexpected things and stimulate new ideas. Perhaps subjective experience is somewhat linked to metacognition, conceptually. Still, a clear theoretical account is needed to tie it all together. But that has to wait until Chapters 7 and 9, I'm afraid.

For now, perhaps it suffices to say that prefrontal lesions and inactivations do not *only* affect perceptual metacognition. Even if one is not convinced yet that perceptual metacognition has anything to do with consciousness, there are independent reasons to think that the prefrontal cortex is causally relevant somehow.

One finding is what I just described in the Section 3.8: Del Cul et al.'s (2009) lesion study. The experiment was not explicitly about metacognition. Unlike Fleming et al.'s (2014) lesion study, the patients were asked to rate subjective visibility rather than confidence. And yet prefrontal lesions impacted these ratings. Also, as I mentioned, there was a small but positive effect on visual discrimination task performance too.

In the olfactory domain, it has been reported a patient with damage to the orbitofrontal cortex suffered the loss of subjective sense of smell, while having preserved automatic responses to pleasant olfactory stimuli (Li et al. 2010).

In other studies, lesions to the prefrontal cortex impaired the patients' visual detection behavior. These patients showed more conservative bias in detection (Colás et al. 2019). That is, they became less likely to report that they saw the stimulus overall, even if their ability to process the stimuli remained intact. Steve Macknik (personal communication) also observed similar patterns of behavior in a patient with damages to the prefrontal cortex. Another study likewise found that patients with lesions to the dorsolateral prefrontal areas were more likely to miss targets in a visual detection task (Barceló, Suwazono, and Knight 2000).

This is consistent with the finding that TMS also impairs other kinds of detection. For example, change blindness refers to the inability to detect changes that occur in one unexpected part of a large visual scene. In general, subjects are not very good with change detection when the change happens simultaneously with other visual transients such as a flash of a blank screen. But detection of changes was made more challenging when magnetic stimulations were administered to both the prefrontal (Turatto, Sandrini, and Miniussi 2004) and parietal cortices (Beck et al. 2006).

In another study, it was found that TMS to the frontal eye fields *enhanced* visual task performance. Again, the task required detection of a simple stimulus, rather than discrimination (Grosbras and Paus 2003).

Lesions to the prefrontal cortex, especially on the right hemisphere, can also lead to spatial neglect, which refers to patients ignoring stimuli on the left (Karnath and Rorden 2012). Again, this somewhat primarily concerns detection, as patients with neglect seem to have implicit knowledge of stimuli presented on the neglected side (Marshall and Halligan 1988). These symptoms are often associated with lesions to the inferior parietal region, but in fact they occur after damages to the prefrontal cortex too. Arguably, these effects may tell us more about attention rather than consciousness per se; the relationship between the two will be addressed in the Chapter 4. However, monkeys with lesions to the frontal eye fields seemed to show genuine deficits in detection, even when only a single stimulus was concerned (Latto and Cowey 1971). Lesions to the dorsolateral prefrontal cortex in monkeys also led to more errors in the detection of a single flash of light (Kamback 1973).

What is special about detection tasks? Arguably, they are very much related to metacognition, as suggested by both computational and empirical modeling studies (Ko and Lau 2012; King and Dehaene 2014; Maniscalco, Peters, and Lau 2016; Peters et al. 2017). They are rather unlike discrimination tasks. In a two-choice discrimination task, we only have to compare the evidence in favor of each option. If there is more evidence in favor of one option over the other, we decide that's the correct answer. In detection, it is far less clear where to draw the line to say there is enough evidence for a "yes" answer. That is because a "no" answer is supposed to be signified by a *lack* of evidence. When we lack evidence, we cannot be certain what is going on. Do we lack evidence because the evidence is not there to be found, or just because *we* failed to find the evidence? And just how little evidence is too little? To decide whether a certain level of evidence is enough for detection, we need to have some idea what counts as enough—*typically for oneself under these situations*. That is to say that successful, unbiased detection requires *self-knowledge*.

The last point is not so straightforward. I hope it will become clearer as we move along (especially in Chapters 7–9). But for now, let us at least be clear that disruptions to prefrontal activity do not *only* impair performance in metacognitive tasks. They affect all sorts of other tasks, especially *detection*, which is arguably very much related to awareness: If one truthfully reports "no I do not see something," contra "yes I see something," it would be odd to say there is surely no difference in subjective experience.

3.10 Direct Stimulation

So far we have focused on the effects of disruption of prefrontal activity: lesions, TMS, and chemical inactivations. But how about direct electric stimulation for the purpose of eliciting activity? Wilder Penfield famously applied this technique to different cortical areas, when patients were going through open-head surgery (1958). It was found that stimulations to the sensory areas (e.g., the visual cortex or somatosensory areas) can elicit spontaneous reports of conscious experiences. Such reports were possible because the patients were kept awake during the surgery; this can help the surgeons map out the functions of the tissues at different locations, via self-reports, to guide the surgery itself.

But what happens when we stimulate the prefrontal cortex? One interesting and well-known finding was about the supplementary motor area, a medial region anterior to the motor cortex. In some cases, when this area was stimulated, patients reported feeling the "urge" to make movements, without actually making them (Fried et al. 1991). This is one of the many reasons why it seems odd to claim that the entire prefrontal cortex isn't constitutively involved in any kind of conscious experience. Certainly, volition, or the experience of motoric intention, is a kind of subjective experience too.

Likewise, stimulation to the orbitofrontal cortex and the anterior cingulate can elicit a wide variety of affective, olfactory, gustatory, and somatosensory experiences (Fox et al. 2018).

But how about other perceptual experiences such as conscious seeing? In particular, the areas concerned here are the lateral and anterior prefrontal regions. Do stimulations to these areas elicit perceptual experiences?

The answer is: rarely, if at all (Raccah, Block, and Fox 2021). There are a few reports that stimulation to the lateral prefrontal areas can elicit spontaneous visual imagery or hallucinations (Bancaud and Talairach 1992; Blanke, Landis, and Seeck 2000; Vignal, Chauvel, and Halgren 2000). But some have argued that these happened only because the stimulation effects spread to early sensory areas. That certainly is possible. Stimulation to an area may have distal effects because brain areas generally do not work in isolation. But once we realize there is such a possibility, how do we know that this did not happen when the early sensory areas were stimulated? How do we know that activity didn't spread to the prefrontal cortex, which ultimately led to the subjective experience?

This issue is not easy to empirically resolve at the moment. The question is not whether stimulating the prefrontal cortex can ever elicit perceptual experiences *at all*. Apparently, it can, at least in some cases. Rather, the right question to ask here may be why is it so much *harder* to elicit such experiences by stimulating the lateral and anterior prefrontal areas compared to the sensory or motor areas? It is admittedly much harder. But the question is why?

One argument could be that some subtle changes in experiences were in fact induced, but the subjects were unable to detect it and to report accordingly. This may sound contrived, but in a way it is exactly what local theorists should accept (Michel and Morales 2019). They claim that the prefrontal cortex is important for attention, access, and report, but not subjective experience per se. So if access is disrupted, there could be unnoticed perceptual changes—a possibility that localists advocate (as we will see in Chapter 4). Independently, we know that disrupting prefrontal activity can lead to detection failures (as reviewed in the Section 3.9), as well as impairment of metacognitive insight (Section 3.5). So this is not an ad hoc assumption.

I suspect though, limitations of current stimulation protocols are also related. The studies discussed here often involve somewhat arbitrarily chosen stimulation intensity and frequency, which we know works for sensory and motor areas. But we know that the physiology of the prefrontal cortex is different. Maybe in the future we need to design new protocols for the prefrontal cortex tailored for matching the dynamic profiles of its activity, given by concurrent recording from the patient tested. Before we can demonstrate that some suitable prefrontal stimulation protocol can abolish perceptual metacognition as measured in the studies by Rounis et al. (2010) and Fleming et al. (2014), perhaps there just isn't much point in debating whether it could elicit vivid perceptual experiences. In those studies, sensitive psychophysical methods were employed to look for subtle effects at near-threshold. If the stimulation just isn't powerful enough to change the relevant measures under those circumstances, it means that the relevant mechanisms just aren't engaged by the stimulation. In this case, naturally we don't expect changes in subjective phenomenology so salient to be spontaneously reported.

Given that the first argument of undetected change in phenomenology already suffices logically as a reply to the localists, why do I emphasize on this second consideration of potentially limited efficacy of stimulation too? Let me explain with the following analogy.

3.11 Pianos and Trumpets

The piano is a beautifully engineered musical instrument. The keys are arranged spatially, so that the lower notes are elicited by the keys on the left and the higher notes on the right. There is a systematic, one-to-one mapping between keys and notes following a clear logic. Just by watching another person play the piano, a total beginner can already appreciate the spatial layout. If the task is to elicit a single sound of a certain pitch, one may have some success figuring it out with a few trial and error attempts. Even toddlers can make some sounds on the piano.

Contrast this with another wonderful instrument, the trumpet. None of the three "buttons" on the instrument uniquely map to a single note. Some notes can be played with different fingerings. Airflow and the "embouchure" are both critical, and yet neither are easily observable by the audience. One would have a hard time figuring out how to play a simple scale just by watching someone else play. Beginners sometimes fail to make any sound at all on first attempts.

But both instruments can make great music. Arguably, one generates the sound more directly when playing the trumpet. On the piano, the keys could have been mapped to the notes in a totally different way, had it been engineered differently. The moral is: the sheer ease of triggering a desired effect does not necessarily tell us the full story of the underlying functions and mechanisms.

The sensory cortices are somewhat like the piano. The visual cortex has a spatial layout known as retinotopy. There is a spatial isomorphism, meaning that two points close in space on the retina tend to trigger activity from neurons that are also spatially close to each other in the visual cortex. So there is in effect a map. This spatial map is also found in the somatosensory areas, where there is a logical and isomorphic representation of the body, sometimes known as the homunculus (a little person) (Figure 3.4). Much of that

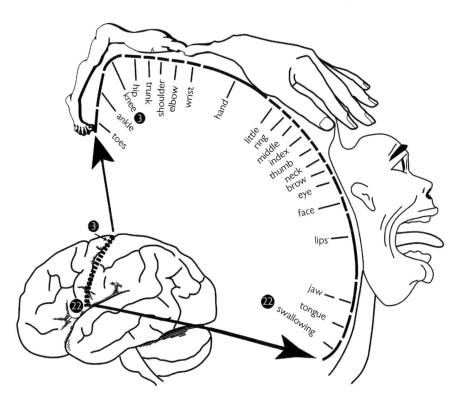

Figure 3.4 Penfield's homunculus: a map of somatosensory representations of different parts of the body in the brain

was detailed in Penfield's work, using the method of direct electric stimulation mentioned in Section 3.10.

Another feature of the sensory cortices is sparse coding, which refers to the fact that at one time, there are relatively few active neurons (Olshausen and Field 2004). To represent something such as an oriented line segment, only a small number of neurons need to fire. This architecture is also sometimes called "labeled lines," as if neurons each carry a label (e.g., "I signal oriented lines at a 42-degree right tilt, for this particular retinal location" or "I signal the face of Barack Obama in a left-facing profile"). This is of course an over-simplification. Things are slightly more complex, where multiple neurons often code similar things, and one neuron is typically involved in multiple representations. But all the same, this describes the basic logic of how things work in the sensory cortices to some extent.

This general pattern very much breaks down in the prefrontal cortex. There, neurons have much larger receptive fields, meaning that they are not so spatially specific. Sometimes they do not concern spatial locations at all. Also, many neurons fire to the same stimuli, only to varying degrees; and the same neuron also seems to respond to many different things (Fusi, Miller, and Rigotti 2016). To read out from the neuronal activity what the subject is perceiving, one often has to aggregate information from many neurons. The lines aren't so clearly "labeled." One needs to use advanced computational methods to "decode" the content (Mante et al. 2013; Rigotti et al. 2013). Instead of providing simple signals for the presence of specific external stimuli, much more complex computations seem to be carried out in the prefrontal cortex.

Now, who wants to complain that learning to play the trumpet is hard? Of course it is, and so is the prefrontal cortex. But we shouldn't write off something just because it is complicated, especially when we are studying something as complicated as consciousness. This is not to say I encourage the reader to accept things which we do not understand either. In Chapters 7 and 9, we will try to understand better the role of the prefrontal cortex in consciousness at a theoretical level.

3.12 Chapter Summary

A famous fable has it that one night a drunk man looked for his keys on the street (Kaplan 1964). Turns out, he lost them in a park far away. When asked why he didn't look for the keys where we lost them, he replied: "But the streetlights are here!"

Vision neuroscientists love the visual cortex. In large part that's because the clear anatomical organization allows for precise physiological measurements to obtain strong experimental effects. Though I too work with vision scientists, I was initially trained in a "prefrontal lab" (Lau et al. 2004). The differences in scientific culture and expectations are often underappreciated. But just because some measurements are more challenging to obtain robustly shouldn't mean we write off the subject altogether. Somebody needs to study the more difficult, messier things.

Here I have given concrete arguments about why criticisms against the role of the prefrontal cortex in consciousness are problematic. They are conceptually unsound, when we reflect on what we really mean by the NCC, and on biological principles such as degeneracy. Given these, we should not expect to find strong effects of disruption of prefrontal activity. Despite these caveats, there is actually considerable positive evidence. These empirical findings are just falsely written off sometimes.

This concludes our first issue, regarding the NCC: the local theorists don't seem to be quite right. But the view that the NCC reflects a global broadcast may also not be entirely convincing either. In Chapter 2 we summarized that the neural signature for subjective experience may be somewhat subtle in the prefrontal cortex. Here we should also concede that the effects of lesions and stimulation are often modest. When they were found, they mostly concerned detection and metacognition. It is true that more salient effects affecting perception in general can be found in the early sensory areas. But those may be due to performance-capacity confounders (see Chapter 2). This is why we continue to pay so much attention to the prefrontal cortex, despite these relatively subtle findings—they are more specific for our purpose of understanding consciousness.

In Chapter 4, we will move on to the next issue, the relationship between attention and consciousness, where we may likewise find an intermediate answer.

References

Alstott J, Breakspear M, Hagmann P et al. Modeling the impact of lesions in the human brain. *PLOS Comput Biol* 2009;5:e1000408.

Bancaud J, Talairach J. Clinical semiology of frontal lobe seizures. *Adv Neurol* 1992;57:3–58.

Barceló F, Suwazono S, Knight RT. Prefrontal modulation of visual processing in humans. *Nat Neurosci* 2000;3:399–403.

Beck DM, Muggleton N, Walsh V et al. Right parietal cortex plays a critical role in change blindness. *Cereb Cortex* 2006;**16**:712–717.

van Bergen RS, Ma WJ, Pratte MS et al. Sensory uncertainty decoded from visual cortex predicts behavior. *Nat Neurosci* 2015;**18**:1728–1730.

Blanke O, Landis T, Seeck M. Electrical cortical stimulation of the human prefrontal cortex evokes complex visual hallucinations. *Epilepsy Behav* 2000;**1**:356–361.

Boly M, Massimini M, Tsuchiya N et al. Are the neural correlates of consciousness in the front or in the back of the cerebral cortex? Clinical and neuroimaging evidence. *J Neurosci* 2017;**37**:9603–9613.

Bor D, Schwartzman DJ, Barrett AB et al. Theta-burst transcranial magnetic stimulation to the prefrontal or parietal cortex does not impair metacognitive visual awareness. *PLOS One* 2017;**12**:e0171793.

Brickner RM. *The Intellectual Functions of the Frontal Lobes: A Study Based Upon Observation of a Man After Partial Bilateral Frontal Lobectomy*. Macmillan, 1936.

Brickner RM. Brain of patient A. after bilateral frontal lobectomy: Status of frontal-lobe problem. *AMA Arch Neurol Psychiatry* 1952;**68**:293–313.

Chiang T-C, Lu R-B, Hsieh S et al. Stimulation in the dorsolateral prefrontal cortex changes subjective evaluation of percepts. *PLOS One* 2014;**9**:e106943.

Colás I, Chica AB, Ródenas E et al. Conscious perception in patients with prefrontal damage. *Neuropsychologia* 2019;**129**:284–293.

Cortese A, Amano K, Koizumi A et al. Multivoxel neurofeedback selectively modulates confidence without changing perceptual performance. *Nat Commun* 2016;**7**:13669.

Croxson PL, Johansen-Berg H, Behrens TEJ et al. Quantitative investigation of connections of the prefrontal cortex in the human and macaque using probabilistic diffusion tractography. *J Neurosci* 2005;**25**:8854–8866.

De Brigard F. Know-how, intellectualism, and memory systems. *Philos Psychol* 2019;**32**:719–758.

Dehaene S. *Consciousness and the Brain: Deciphering How the Brain Codes Our Thoughts*. Penguin, 2014.

Del Cul A, Dehaene S, Reyes P et al. Causal role of prefrontal cortex in the threshold for access to consciousness. *Brain* 2009;**132**:2531–2540.

Fleming SM, Ryu J, Golfinos JG et al. Domain-specific impairment in metacognitive accuracy following anterior prefrontal lesions. *Brain* 2014;**137**:2811–2822.

Fleming SM, Weil RS, Nagy Z et al. Relating introspective accuracy to individual differences in brain structure. *Science* 2010;**329**:1541–1543.

Fox KCR, Yih J, Raccah O et al. Changes in subjective experience elicited by direct stimulation of the human orbitofrontal cortex. *Neurology* 2018;**91**:e1519–e1527.

Fried I, Katz A, McCarthy G et al. Functional organization of human supplementary motor cortex studied by electrical stimulation. *J Neurosci* 1991;**11**:3656–3666.

Fusi S, Miller EK, Rigotti M. Why neurons mix: High dimensionality for higher cognition. *Curr Opin Neurobiol* 2016;**37**:66–74.

Gazzaniga MS. *The Cognitive Neurosciences*. MIT Press, 2009.

Grosbras M-H, Paus T. Transcranial magnetic stimulation of the human frontal eye field facilitates visual awareness. *Eur J Neurosci* 2003;**18**:3121–3126.

Huang Y-Z, Edwards MJ, Rounis E et al. Theta burst stimulation of the human motor cortex. *Neuron* 2005;**45**:201–206.

Jonas E, Kording KP. Could a neuroscientist understand a microprocessor? *PLOS Comput Biol* 2017;**13**:e1005268.

Kamback MC. Detection of brief light flashes by monkeys (Macaca nemestrina) with dorsolateral frontal ablations. *Neuropsychologia* 1973;**11**:325–329.

Kandel E. *Principles of Neural Science*, fifth edition. McGraw Hill Professional, 2013.

Kaplan A. *The Conduct of Inquiry: Methodology for Behavioral Science*. Routledge, 1964.

Karnath H-O, Rorden C. The anatomy of spatial neglect. *Neuropsychologia* 2012;**50**:1010–1017.

Katsuki F. Unique and shared roles of the posterior parietal and dorsolateral prefrontal cortex in cognitive functions. *Front Integr Neurosci* 2012;**6**. https://doi.org/10.3389/fnint.2012.00017.

King J-R, Dehaene S. A model of subjective report and objective discrimination as categorical decisions in a vast representational space. *Philos Trans R Soc Lond B Biol Sci* 2014;**369**:20130204.

Koch C. What is consciousness? *Nature* 2018;**557**:S8–S12.

Koch C, Massimini M, Boly M et al. Neural correlates of consciousness: progress and problems. *Nat Rev Neurosci* 2016;**17**:307–321.

Ko Y, Lau H. A detection theoretic explanation of blindsight suggests a link between conscious perception and metacognition. *Philos Trans R Soc Lond B Biol Sci* 2012;**367**:1401–1411.

Lak A, Costa GM, Romberg E et al. Orbitofrontal cortex is required for optimal waiting based on decision confidence. *Neuron* 2014;**84**:190–201.

Lapate RC, Samaha J, Rokers B et al. Perceptual metacognition of human faces is causally supported by function of the lateral prefrontal cortex. *Commun Biol* 2019;**3**:360. https://doi.org/10.1038/s42003-020-1049-3.

Latto R, Cowey A. Visual field defects after frontal eye-field lesions in monkeys. *Brain Res* 1971;**30**:1–24.

Lau HC, Rogers RD, Ramnani N et al. Willed action and attention to the selection of action. *Neuroimage* 2004;**21**:1407–1415.

Lim S, Hutchings F, Kaiser M. Modeling the impact of lesions in the brain. In: Ooyen AV, Butz-Ostendorf M eds. *The Rewiring Brain* Academic Press, 2017:465–484.

Li W, Lopez L, Osher J et al. Right orbitofrontal cortex mediates conscious olfactory perception. *Psychol Sci* 2010;**21**:1454–1463.

Maniscalco B, Lau H. A signal detection theoretic approach for estimating metacognitive sensitivity from confidence ratings. *Conscious Cogn* 2012;**21**:422–430.

Maniscalco B, Lau H. The signal processing architecture underlying subjective reports of sensory awareness. *Neurosci Conscious* 2016;**2016**. https://doi.org/10.1093/nc/niw002.

Maniscalco B, Peters MAK, Lau H. Heuristic use of perceptual evidence leads to dissociation between performance and metacognitive sensitivity. *Atten Percept Psychophys* 2016;**78**:923–937.

Mante V, Sussillo D, Shenoy KV et al. Context-dependent computation by recurrent dynamics in prefrontal cortex. *Nature* 2013;**503**:78–84.

Marshall JC, Halligan PW. Blindsight and insight in visuo-spatial neglect. *Nature* 1988;**336**:766–767.

Mashour GA, Roelfsema P, Changeux J-P et al. Conscious processing and the global neuronal workspace hypothesis. *Neuron* 2020;**105**:776–798.

Mason PH. Degeneracy at multiple levels of complexity. *Biol Theory* 2010;**5**:277–288.

Ma WJ, Beck JM, Latham PE et al. Bayesian inference with probabilistic population codes. *Nat Neurosci* 2006;**9**:1432–1438.

McCurdy LY, Maniscalco B, Metcalfe J et al. Anatomical coupling between distinct metacognitive systems for memory and visual perception. *J Neurosci* 2013;**33**:1897–1906.

Metcalfe J, Son LK. Anoetic, noetic, and autonoetic metacognition. In: Beran MJ, Brandl J, Perner J, Proust J eds. *Foundations of Metacognition.* OUP Oxford, 2012:289–301.

Michel M, Morales J. Minority reports: Consciousness and the prefrontal cortex. *Mind Lang* 2019;**35**(4):493-513. https://doi.org/10.1111/mila.12264.

Miyamoto K, Osada T, Setsuie R et al. Causal neural network of metamemory for retrospection in primates. *Science* 2017;**355**:188–193.

Miyamoto K, Trudel N, Kamermans K et al. Identification and disruption of a neural mechanism for accumulating prospective metacognitive information prior to decision-making. *Neuron* 2021;**0**. https://doi.org/10.1016/j.neuron.2021.02.024.

Musso M, Moro A, Glauche V et al. Broca's area and the language instinct. *Nat Neurosci* 2003;**6**:774–781.

Nakamura RK, Mishkin M. Chronic "blindness" following lesions of nonvisual cortex in the monkey. *Exp Brain Res* 1986;**63**:173–184.

Odegaard B, Knight RT, Lau H. Should a few null findings falsify prefrontal theories of conscious perception? *J Neurosci* 2017;**37**:9593–9602.

Olshausen B, Field D. Sparse coding of sensory inputs. *Curr Opin Neurobiol* 2004;**14**:481–487.

Penfield W. Some mechanisms of consciousness discovered during electrical stimulation of the brain. *Proc Natl Acad Sci U S A* 1958;**44**:51–66.

Peters MAK, Ro T, Lau H. Who's afraid of response bias? *Neurosci Conscious* 2016;**2016**:niw001.

Peters MAK, Thesen T, Ko YD et al. Perceptual confidence neglects decision-incongruent evidence in the brain. *Nat Hum Behav* 2017;**1**. https://doi.org/10.1038/s41 562-017-0139.

Petrides M, Pandya DN. Association pathways of the prefrontal cortex and functional observations. In: Stuss DJ, Knight RT eds. *Principles of Frontal Lobe Function*; OUP Oxford, 2002:31–50.

Pollen DA. Fundamental requirements for primary visual perception. *Cereb Cortex* 2008;**18**:1991–1998.

Raccah O, Block N, Fox KCR. Does the prefrontal cortex play an essential role in consciousness? Insights from intracranial electrical stimulation of the human brain. *J Neurosci* 2021;**41**:2076–2087.

Rahnev D, Nee DE, Riddle J et al. Causal evidence for frontal cortex organization for perceptual decision making. *Proc Natl Acad Sci U S A* 2016;**113**:6059–6064.

Rhodes MG, Castel AD. Metacognitive illusions for auditory information: effects on monitoring and control. *Psychon Bull Rev* 2009;**16**:550–554.

Richter FR, Cooper RA, Bays PM et al. Distinct neural mechanisms underlie the success, precision, and vividness of episodic memory. *Elife* 2016;**5**. https://doi.org/ 10.7554/eLife.18260.

Rigotti M, Barak O, Warden MR et al. The importance of mixed selectivity in complex cognitive tasks. *Nature* 2013;**497**:585–590.

Rounis E, Maniscalco B, Rothwell JC et al. Theta-burst transcranial magnetic stimulation to the prefrontal cortex impairs metacognitive visual awareness. *Cogn Neurosci* 2010;**1**:165–175.

Ruby E, Maniscalco B, Peters MAK. On a "failed" attempt to manipulate visual metacognition with transcranial magnetic stimulation to prefrontal cortex. *Conscious Cogn* 2018;**62**:34–41.

Stanley J, Krakauer JW. Motor skill depends on knowledge of facts. *Front Hum Neurosci* 2013;**7**:503.

Tononi G, Sporns O, Edelman GM. Measures of degeneracy and redundancy in biological networks. *Proc Natl Acad Sci U S A* 1999;**96**:3257–3262.

Turatto M, Sandrini M, Miniussi C. The role of the right dorsolateral prefrontal cortex in visual change awareness. *Neuroreport* 2004;**15**:2549–2552.

Vignal JP, Chauvel P, Halgren E. Localised face processing by the human prefrontal cortex: Stimulation-evoked hallucinations of faces. *Cogn Neuropsychol* 2000;**17**:281–291.

Voytek B, Davis M, Yago E et al. Dynamic neuroplasticity after human prefrontal cortex damage. *Neuron* 2010;**68**:401–408.

Walker EY, Cotton RJ, Ma WJ et al. A neural basis of probabilistic computation in visual cortex. *Nat Neurosci* 2020;**23**:122–129.

Ye Q, Zou F, Lau H et al. Causal evidence for mnemonic metacognition in human precuneus. *J Neurosci* 2018;**38**:6379–6387.

Yonelinas AP, Aly M, Wang W-C et al. Recollection and familiarity: Examining controversial assumptions and new directions. *Hippocampus* 2010;**20**:1178–1194.

4

Untouched Raw Feels?

4.1 Speckled Hen

A well-known philosophical puzzle concerns a speckled hen (Chisholm 1942). Imagine looking at one. Within just half a second, you can probably already see that the bird is speckled. Let's say you close your eyes from there. If I ask you to describe the speckle pattern, you may be able to say: it is lightly speckled, somewhat regular. Perhaps it is less speckled than another bird you just saw earlier. The pattern is somewhat even. There's not a missing patch in one particular place.

So you seem to have perceived a fair bit of detail. But did you see every single speckle? That seems improbable. You didn't attentively *look* at every speckle, as if you were counting them. That would have taken much longer than half a second. But if you saw the hen as evenly covered in speckles, perhaps you didn't *miss* any speckle either. So let's pick a particular speckle. Did you see it or not? Can you answer that question with any degree of certainty?

There are very many variants of this puzzle, and they have exercised the imagination of philosophers and scientists alike for centuries. As in the problem of the neural correlates of consciousness, Matthias Michel conducted a masterful review of the historical literature (2019), tracing the origin of the puzzle back to the nineteenth century.

The puzzle concerns the relationship between attention and the subjective experience of perception. Do we need to attentively look at something to have a subjective experience of seeing it? Or can subjective experience occur without us even *noticing* the relevant events?

This is the second of the five core issues outlined in Chapter 1. As you will see, our answer to this question may not be as conclusive as our answer to the first issue. Fortunately, what we have already learned from the first issue may ultimately inform us here.

In Consciousness We Trust. Hakwan Lau, Oxford University Press. © Hakwan Lau 2022.
DOI: 10.1093/oso/9780198856771.003.0005

4.2 Iconic Memory

In the modern empirical literature, many relevant experiments employ Sperling's "post-cue" procedure (1960). In this kind of experiment, we usually present an array of 12 letters to subjects, organized as three rows of four letters each. Let's say we only flash these 12 letters on the screen for half a second. If we ask subjects to report all the letters, they can probably only get the first few right. But it would be premature to conclude that subjects can only see a few letters, rather than all 12. That's because, even if all of the letters are recognized during the presentation, subjects may be already forgetting some letters while reporting the first few. In other words, the bottleneck may be reporting and memory, rather than seeing.

So Sperling (1960) presented a tone right *after* the letters disappeared, to tell the subjects which row of letters they had to report. A high pitch meant that subjects had to report the top row, a middle pitch the middle row, and a low pitch the bottom row. This way, subjects could do the task almost perfectly: they could often report all four letters correctly, in *any* of the rows post-cued. This suggests that reporting and memory are indeed the bottleneck. Most of the 12 letters, rather than just a few, were visually processed in the brain, even at this brief presentation (Figure 4.1).

One interpretation would be: this supports the local view. According to the view, subjective experiences arise at some early high-capacity stage, possibly locally within the early visual areas. So that stage may have all 12 recognized letters represented. Attention only limits the capacity for late-stage read out. Without directing our selective attention with post-cuing to a particular row, we cannot report *all* of the letters in the array. But, all the same, all 12 letters were at some point consciously represented. Ned Block describes this interpretation as phenomenological overflow (2007). That is, our subjective experience is richer in details than what we can cognitively access.

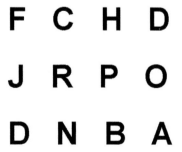

Figure 4.1 An example array of 12 letters presented in the Sperling experiments

However, this is not the standard interpretation of these findings in vision science, and perhaps for good reasons. Sperling himself (1960) was careful to call the putative early stage high-capacity storage "iconic memory," without stipulating so strongly that it has to be conscious. As we have learned from the previous chapters, one lesson from blindsight is that being able to report certain visual content does not necessarily imply consciousness. What the Sperling experiments showed is that we have the relevant information for all 12 letters represented briefly. But this doesn't necessarily mean we consciously saw them all in detail.

Indeed, there is some evidence that if we replace some letters in an uncued row with some non-letter symbols, subjects may not notice (de Gardelle, Sackur, and Kouider 2009). So the global theorists can very well argue that the subjects only consciously saw 12 letter-like symbols arranged on a 4 × 3 grid. The conscious recognition of specific letters may only happen at the time of post-cuing, and only for the specific row cued. But as we will discuss next, this view runs into problems too. So this debate is very much ongoing.

4.3 Is Attention "Necessary"?

It may be tempting to formulate the debate as one about whether attention is *necessary* for consciousness. In these terms, the global theorists say that attention is necessary, which the local theorists deny. This is more or less right. The global theorists deny that we consciously see all 12 letters as specific recognized letters, or every single speckle on the hen individually. That's because within a brief presentation we do not have time to attentively look at them one-by-one. Without attention, early sensory information may not be able to enter the central workspace and, therefore, remains nonconscious. The local theorists maintain that attention is only needed for reporting or cognitive access, but not for subjective experience to arise.

But by now the reader should be aware that the notion of "necessity," as applied to cognitive neuroscience experiments, is often misleading and confusing (see Sections 2.3, 2.4, 3.2, and 3.11). Some relevant experimental findings may help to drive this point home.

In Ulric Neisser's classic experiments on the phenomenon of "selective looking" (Neisser and Becklen 1975), subjects were told to pay attention to some specific events, like the number of times some players pass the basketball to their teammate (wearing the same jersey). While the basketball "game" was happening, irrelevant but noteworthy events could happen, such as a person holding an open umbrella walking slowly through the scene. Many subjects entirely missed these surprising events, as they were absorbed in counting basketball passes. There are many variants of this phenomenon, some famously involving a person in a gorilla suit doing a wiggle dance, rather than a person holding an umbrella (Chabris and Simons 2010). These are also sometimes called inattentional blindness experiments.

On the face of it, these findings may seem to support the global view. That is, when attention is directed elsewhere, one seems to be completely unable to notice these remarkable events. But the localists can point out that not all subjects missed the events. Also these may be exceptional situations. There may be some other tasks where the subjects were able to detect some events in the periphery while they were also occupied by the main task (Li et al. 2002). So, attention may be needed for some subjects, in some situations, to detect some stimuli. But not always. Attention is, therefore, not strictly necessary.

But how do we know whether the subjects' attention was sufficiently occupied by the central task, in any of these cases? The trouble is, attention, like many constructs in cognitive neuroscience, is not directly measurable. Therefore, the strategy of trying to occupy it *completely* to test for necessity may not be as straightforward as it seems. This is not to say these findings are anything short of amazing. But for the purpose of arbitrating between the global and local views, we may also need to consider the relationship between attention and subjective perception in more general terms.

4.4 Load Theory

Concerning the general relationship between task demand and perception, few ideas are as relevant and important as Nili Lavie's Load Theory of Attention (2005).

Over half a century ago, at the beginning of cognitive science, there was a classic debate on the role of attention in perception (Driver 2001). The early selectionists held that attention acts like a filter, blocking out unattended stimuli before their meanings are processed. That is, the simple physical properties of a stimulus, like the volume or pitch of a sound, may be preattentively processed. But to understand the meaning of an utterance, or the identity of a word or letter, we need to pay attention. The late selectionists, on the other hand, said that unattended stimuli are also processed at deep levels. When subjects fail to report certain unattended stimuli, the late selectionists argued it may be a failure of memory rather than perception.

Lavie's load theory beautifully resolved the debate. The idea is that our brain adopts different selection strategies depending on perceptual demand. When the perceptual task at hand is difficult, such as having to make decisions based upon multiple features of a stimulus rather than detection of a single feature, we are said to be under high perceptual load. Under such high perceptual load, naturally, the brain needs to filter stimuli out early to avoid congestion. On the other hand, under low perceptual load, the brain may adopt a late selection strategy, because it can afford to do so.

Much of the supporting evidence for Load Theory comes from behavioral studies (Lavie 2005). But in some experiments, functional magnetic resonance imaging (fMRI) was employed to assess how perceptual load at a central task may impact the processing of some peripheral, task-irrelevant stimuli (Schwartz et al. 2005). As predicted by the theory, under high load, there was less brain activity associated with the processing of task-irrelevant stimuli, as if such stimuli were filtered out early on. Interestingly, this effect was observed as early as in V1 (the primary visual cortex), where neurons respond to specific orientations of line segments, among other low-level features. This means that when the perceptual task is challenging enough, attentional filtering may happen even earlier than early selectionists suggested. It seems to take place before the processing of "meaning," as object identity is typically thought to be represented in area IT (inferotemporal cortex), well after V1 processing.

4.5 Post-Cuing Impacts Early Sensory Activity

To put this back into the context of Sperling's post-cue experiments, we can consider some elegant findings by Claire Sergent and colleagues (2011). These experiments employed a similar post-cue procedure. But instead of using letters as stimuli, the authors presented some simple abstract stimuli known as Gabor patches (see Chapter 2, Figure 2.1). The processing of these stimuli is reflected by activity in early visual areas, such as V1 and V2 (another early visual area).

The subjects had to report the orientation of these Gabor patches. Post-cuing improved task performance, as expected. Critically, the authors also found that post-cuing modulated activity in V1 and V2. That is, for early visual regions that are specific to the retinotopic location of a Gabor patch, there was more activity when the relevant Gabor patch was post-cued, as compared to when some other Gabor patch in a different location was post-cued. One may wonder: does this mean that the activity for post-cued stimulus was enhanced, or the activity for uncued stimulus was reduced? The answer is probably both. Given the ubiquitous nature of lateral competition within a cortical circuit, when some activity is enhanced, the nearby activity tends to be damp-ened (Carandini and Heeger 2011).

This seems to make the simple story favored by local theorists rather im-plausible. The story is that there is a high-capacity storage mechanism in early sensory areas. Attention does not change its activity, but only limits its readout by a late-stage, low-capacity access mechanism. So if subjective ex-perience happens in these early sensory areas, attention is not that important. But trouble is, attention actually changes these early activities, measurable in direct neuronal recordings too (Treue 2001).

Perhaps the localist can argue that these changes in visual activity by atten-tion are not essential for subjective experience. They only happen after the conscious recognition of the stimuli. But together with the evidence in sup-port of Load Theory reviewed in the Section 4.4, this seems somewhat un-likely. These attentional gating effects on early sensory areas seem functionally important for perception itself. Also, because of the phenomenon of lateral competition mentioned earlier, it is likely that after post-cuing, the uncued stimuli are no longer accessible—all due to local competition with the visual areas rather than late-stage access limitations in, for example, the prefrontal cortex.

4.6 Apparent Richness

So, some problems with the local view have now been highlighted. But the global view is not so appealing either, especially regarding how it can accom-modate the phenomenology of perception. In part, the problem is that atten-tion is known to have a limited bandwidth (He, Cavanagh, and Intriligator 1996). If attention is the bottleneck for information entering consciousness, as global theorists suggest, it would be hard to account for the apparent richness of experience.

This point can be appreciated when we consider cases of "selective looking" (i.e., inattentional blindness). Suppose we are one of those subjects who missed the person carrying an opened umbrella, or the gorilla. Our attention is supposed to be focused almost entirely on the basketball passes. And yet, the background at no point looks as if it fades out. Instead, it *seems* to be there, rich and stable—that is why missing the gorilla is so surprising to us. Just how do we account for that appearance of richness? This is a real problem because when it comes to subjective experience, how it *seems* matters.

Local theorists appeal to this richness of appearance too. Block argues that this subjective richness is supported by anecdotal reports from subjects. In turn this "meshes" with the high capacity of early sensory processing (Block 2007). Turns out, these self-reports on subjective richness are far from universal. When asked systematically, many subjects did not report the kind of richness described by local theorists (Cova, Gaillard, and Kammerer 2020).

But let us grant the localists the point that *some* subjects may indeed find perception to be subjectively rich. The problem is that even for these subjects, early sensory representations are modulated strongly by attention, as pointed out earlier in Sections 4.4 and 4.5. Even when you are attending to the same spatial location, these representations are modulated by perceptual load. But to the extent that one claims to have a subjective impression of richness, this impression seems relatively *stable*. A subtle change in the perceptual task does not seem to change this overall impression so much. And yet the early sensory activities are known to change reliably. In this sense, Block's "mesh" argument may actually backfire.

4.7 Too Much Overflow

The last point about backfiring can be further illustrated by a study conducted by the local theorists themselves (Sligte et al. 2010). In the original Sperling experiment, the post-cue was effective up until about half a second after the stimulus array disappeared. Experiments from Lamme's lab have often reported longer effective periods for post-cuing (Landman, Spekreijse, and Lamme 2003). This is likely because they cleverly modified the task into change detection. So in these studies, there was a first array of some items. After a delay, another array was presented, in which one of the items might have changed. Instead of reporting the identities of the items, the subjects only had to report whether there was a change of items between the two arrays in a specific location (indicated by a spatial post-cue *not* shown in Figure 4.2). Under this setup, the post-cue, presented after the offset of the first array, tended to be effective for longer, up to a whole second or more before the onset of the second array.

But a successful detection of change does not necessarily mean that one consciously saw the item in the first array. It could be driven by a hunch that the item in the second array looked somewhat novel, or that there might be some hint of motion or flicker between the arrays. To verify that, Sligte et al. (2010) presented four items to the subjects after there was a change, and asked subjects to identify which one was the prechange item from the first array (Figure 4.2.). A correct identification would indicate that the subject saw the prechange item with at least some detail at "high resolution." Based on the

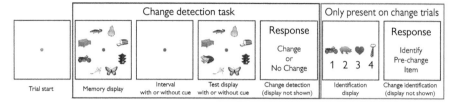

Figure 4.2 The change detection task used by Sligte et al (2010)

Reproduced from Sligte IG, Vandenbroucke ARE, Scholte HS and Lamme VAF (2010) Detailed sensory memory, sloppy working memory. *Front. Psychology* 1:175. doi: 10.3389/fpsyg.2010.00175. This is an open-access article subject to an exclusive license agreement between the authors and the Frontiers Research Foundation

subjects' performance levels, Sligte et al. calculated that "most" items (71%) post-cued in the way described above were perceived at this high resolution.

One could still quibble about the logic of this claim of "high-resolution" perception. Perhaps one does not have to see the prechange item (i.e., from the first array) so clearly to distinguish it from three other items, especially if the items were colorful. Sligte et al. took care to address this point and reported that for gray-scale-only items, successful postchange identification was at 68.8%. One could further argue that even low-resolution perception could support some level of above-chance performance in this four-choice discrimination task. But overall, many have found this to be convincing evidence for perceptual richness in this task; as of 2021, the paper has been cited over 100 times.

Unfortunately, it turns out there was a simple error in Sligte et al.'s calculation. The details are probably not important, but for those who are interested: the authors calculated the number of items perceived at "high resolution" by first calculating Cowan's K (Cowan 2001) for the change detection task (i.e., the average number of items for which a change can be successfully detected), and then multiplying this number by the percent correct score on the prechange identification task. The error here is in not taking into account the fact that chance performance on a four-alternative forced choice (4AFC) task is 25%. Therefore, by their calculation, even chance performance on the prechange identification task would yield a nonzero capacity for the number of high-resolution items. This error can be roughly corrected by normalizing prechange identification percent correct scores by subtracting 25% and dividing by 75%, and then multiplying the resulting normalized score by Cowan's K on the change detection task.

If we correct for that error, the percentage of items supposedly perceived at "high resolution" was only 58.4% for gray-scale items. This is close to what they previously reported (erroneously, from the same error) as the percentage for ordinary working memory (55.0%), assessed in a similar condition without post-cue between the arrays. Prior to the realization of that error, the authors described this range of performance as "sloppy" (from the very title of the article).

So, is the conscious perception of the briefly presented array of items actually "sloppy"? Or is it so rich that it apparently overflows access? Simple errors of the kind made by Sligte et al. are not uncommon in science. My intention here is not to be petty about what is clearly an honest mistake; I myself have no doubt made a countless number of them. But the point is, local theorists have accepted the logic and interpretation of these experiments. If they found the previously reported findings to be exactly congruent with their subjective impression, then this error means that their impression was actually *incompatible* with the data.

4.8　Summary Statistics and Peripheral Vision

In addressing this problem of apparent richness, one solution favored by some global theorists is to think of our representation of the unattended background as a summary (Cohen, Dennett, and Kanwisher 2016). So, instead of representing individual trees in a natural scene background, one may just represent something like: "a bunch of trees of a certain type." Obviously, this does not have to be in the form of a noun phrase as used in natural language. It may contain quantitative information representing the statistics too (e.g., roughly how many trees, the average size, variance, and spatial frequencies of the image). Or it can capture the "gist" of the scene, invoking some complex schematic representations. In fact, this is more than just an idea. This is an active area of vision research with ample empirical support (Alvarez 2011; Rosenholtz 2020).

This is likely how we actually represent things outside of our attentional focus. But it is not clear how this reflects the phenomenology. Some readers may find it odd, too, to think that we consciously see the unattended background as some summary statistics or a gist. At least that isn't introspectively obvious. Instead, some of us may *feel* that one sees the visual world as relatively uniform with details. Perhaps we don't actually represent those details in a picturesque fashion. But all the same, we need an account for why at least some naive subjects feel they do.

This is not to deny that central foveal vision—usually our focus of attention—is subjectively clearer and more vivid. But as one moves away from the fovea toward the visual periphery, the gradient does not seem to fall off as dramatically as the anatomy and physiology of early vision would suggest. Recall from our middle school biology class that the color-sensitive cone cells on the retina are mostly concentrated around the foveal area. And most of our early vision neurons also have receptive fields around the central region. As we move into the periphery, the receptive fields get larger. Roughly, this means our spatial resolution is poorer there. Of course we have *some* color sensitivity and spatial resolution in the periphery. But empirically we seem far poorer than we intuitively think we are (Cohen, Botch, and Robertson 2020).

This seems to create a difficult challenge for both local and global theorists. We just don't seem to have as much visual detail as we feel we have—perhaps anywhere in the brain—because it is missing from the very beginning, sometimes as early as from the retinal level.

Some localists have argued that the paucity of color vision in the periphery may be exaggerated. For example, Block (2019) cited the fact that if we enlarge the stimulus for the periphery, it would look just as colorful as the central stimuli (Tyler 2015). But trouble is, in everyday life, things don't enlarge themselves for our convenience as they enter our peripheral vision. So for a normal, natural stimulus of a constant size, its color would be harder to discern as it moves away from our fovea. And yet, the ordinary, untrained observer tends not to be fully aware of this limitation.

4.9 Inflation

Perhaps the answer to the puzzle of apparent richness is that the details are never represented as such—neither in explicit nor compressed summary forms. Instead, we just *interpret* the sensory representations *as if* they are rich in detail, even when they are not (Knotts et al. 2019). This may not be such a misleading kind of misinterpretation in the end, because the details are actually out there in the world, often just one shift of gaze or attentional focus away. So this may be somewhat like the light inside the refrigerator: because whenever we check it, it is on, we may mistakenly think it is always on (Kouider, de Gardelle, and Dupoux 2007). We can call this an *inflation* account. That is, the richness of a perceptual representation may be overinterpreted or somehow exaggerated at a later stage.

When I say "we" interpret the sensory representation, I do not really mean that we, as people, have to decide to do this with effort. Instead I am referring to some subpersonal, automatic mechanism that is an integral part of the perceptual process itself. This is congruent with the long-standing view in vision science that there is always a decision-making component in perception. It is also true that a person can make postperceptual decisions based on what one learns from perception; I can see an apple and decide to not report it as an apple. But here perceptual decision-making refers to what is part of perception itself. Suppose some neurons are firing in your primary visual cortex. Some process is needed to decide what the neuronal activity really represents: it could be baseline noise, or it could reflect a meaningful signal. Without this process, perception just isn't complete. Inflation is hypothesized to take place at this level of subpersonal perceptual decision-making.

Likewise, inflation can happen at the perceptual metacognitive level too. But this is again not to be confused with the kind of metacognition that involves a person explicitly trying to think about oneself and one's thoughts. It refers to the automatic, subpersonal process of monitoring how well a certain perceptual process has gone. The selective looking (i.e., inattentional blindness) examples help illustrate this point. When we miss the unexpected events, we not only miss it but are also extremely surprised. That's because, based on the perceptual experience itself, we fully expect to be able to see such events. This expectation seems to be formed automatically. Without much effort of introspection, we already "think" we see more than we really do. Perhaps inflation takes place at this subpersonal level too.

There is a fair bit of empirical evidence to support the inflation account. At the perceptual decision-making level, subjects detect stimuli at a less attended spatial location with a more liberal bias. Surprisingly, this happens even when sensitivity for the attended and unattended locations were matched. That is, under relative lack of attention they say they see the stimulus more often, leading to more hits (correct detection), as well as false alarms (apparent "hallucinations," i.e., alleged detection when the stimulus was not really there). This phenomenon was discovered by Dobromir Rahnev, when he was a graduate student in my lab (Rahnev et al. 2011). Brian Odegaard and others followed it up, and found that it replicates robustly and generalizes to more complex and naturalistic stimuli too (Li, Lau, and Odegaard 2018; Odegaard et al. 2018).

These findings suggest some compensatory mechanisms on the subjective level, "inflating" the typically weaker sensitivity associated with the lack of spatial attention. Under the lack of attention, they treated the signal as present even when it wasn't particularly strong. This is true when we compared central versus peripheral vision too. Together with others, another former postdoc fellow in my lab, Guillermo Solovey, found that peripheral vision was associated with more liberal detection, compared to central vision (Solovey, Graney, and Lau 2015).

At the level of perceptual metacognition, stimuli presented at less attended spatial locations also led to higher visibility ratings (Rahnev et al. 2011), even though they were not better discriminated (i.e., again, matched sensitivity). Another piece of evidence concerns crowding, which occurs outside of central vision (Pelli and Tillman 2008). When a perfectly visible stimulus, such as a single letter presented at the periphery, is flanked closely by other stimuli, we may have trouble seeing it. This partly explains why reading in the periphery is close to impossible. Under crowding, subjects seemed overconfident, especially for incorrect trials (Odegaard et al. 2018).

Overall, these empirical findings support the intuition that people seem to generally overestimate how much they see in inattentional blindness and change blindness studies. These intuitions have also been confirmed in studies using questionnaires (Levin and Angelone 2008).

4.10 Limitations of Inflation

I am in favor of this inflation account because I feel that neither the global nor local theories can ultimately account for the apparent richness of subjective experience. The issue is that such richness may not be "real." Some of the details may not actually be represented anywhere in the brain. So fighting over whether such representations are local or global may turn out to be futile. Instead, what we need is a mechanistic account of the *appearance* of stable richness, despite its lack of actually rich content.

But I must acknowledge, the inflation account isn't fully developed, and it has several limitations. The first is that empirical evidence at the level of metacognition is somewhat weak. Besides the reported few cases in Section 4.9, I confess there have also been at least several cases of null results from my own laboratory. Others have even found the opposite results (Zizlsperger, Sauvigny, and Haarmeier 2012; Toscani, Mamassian, and Valsecchi 2021). One possibility is that this kind of effect may only be found for visibility ratings, but not commonly for confidence, as has been suggested by a certain model (King and Dehaene 2014). But also relevant is the fact that in psychophysics experiments, subjects do very many repetitions (i.e., trials) of the same perceptual exercise. Throughout the course they may learn to calibrate their confidence. Even in the absence of feedback, the sheer exercise of repetitive introspection may be sufficient to wipe out the natural tendency to show inflation in metacognitive judgments.

Does it mean the inflation effect isn't real because it is only there for the "untrained" subjects, with their "unreflected" minds? I don't think so.

Instead this may be a reminder that the intuitions of academics on this subject may well be very biased. Many of us have been reflecting on this for decades, and some of us have routinely participated in our own experiments. We may have long forgotten what it was once like. In this sense, questionnaire answers from a large group of untrained subjects may be more meaningful. And as mentioned earlier, they do support inflation (Levin and Angelone 2008).

Incidentally, the evidence at the level of simple perceptual decision-making (i.e., detection bias) is strong. It's been replicated many times, under rather different conditions (Rahnev et al. 2011; Li, Lau, and Odegaard 2018; Odegaard et al. 2018). Perhaps the reason is, when the question wasn't explicitly metacognitive in nature (concerning confidence), they focused less on calibrating their answers, and just reported how the stimulus looked to them.

Some have argued that this kind of detection bias only reflects cognition or responding strategies (Abid 2019). It is unfortunate that this remains a common misunderstanding: to see bias effects as *necessarily* cognitive and postperceptual. In part there might have been historical reasons (Witt et al. 2015; Peters, Ro and Lau 2016). But in fact, many clearly perceptual phenomena show up as effects of biases rather than sensitivity alone (Polat and Sagi 2007; Grove et al. 2012; Meyerhoff and Scholl 2018). See also Michel and Lau (2021) for a review.

It is also true that *sometimes* bias effects are actually uninteresting. If I threaten you and tell you not to say you see anything, and reward you generously for obliging, there's no doubt that this could make you respond more conservatively (i.e., opposite of liberal) without actually changing your visual experience. But in experiments we can carefully rule out such possibilities. For the results reviewed for inflation, some were obtained after considerable training and feedback (Rahnev et al. 2011; Solovey, Graney, and Lau 2015). Subjects were repetitively informed if they were being too liberal for the unattended, and in some cases monetarily incentivized to be neither. The persistence of the liberal biases suggests rather strongly that they were not cognitive. Instead, they likely reflect what people actually consciously saw.

In any case, effects congruent with the inflation account have been demonstrated in other ways too. For example, Valsecchi et al (2018) asked subjects to adjust the stimuli on the screen by pressing keys to match the subjective sharpness of the edges of a pair of stimuli: one presented centrally and one peripherally. Using this matching method, more physical sharpness was required for the central stimulus to appear as sharp as the peripheral one. This means that subjects saw the peripheral stimuli as more sharp and less distorted, subjectively.

Finally, one may have the impression that inflation goes against some well-known findings from Marisa Carrasco's lab (2011). In many experiments, it's been reported that attention boosted the appearance of the stimulus, making it appear to have a higher luminance contrast, for example. Although some of these findings are in dispute (Beck and Schneider 2017), I am inclined to believe that the phenomenon is real. But it does not go against the inflation account, because the inflation effects typically concern the appearance of the stimulus *when* stimulus sensitivity is matched (between the attended and less attended). Under attention, sensitivity is typically boosted. Carrasco's experiments found that under such boosted sensitivity, appearance was boosted too. This is just as expected, assuming stronger perceptual signals should have some positive impact on appearance.

In fact, such effects of appearance boosting by attention may have been partially cancelled out by the inflation mechanisms. This would account for why the effects may be subtle, and therefore controversial at times. Importantly, however, this may reflect cooperation rather than competition. As William James put it (1910), attention makes a perceptual experience more intense, but regarding the true nature of the stimulus "it seems never to lead [our] judgment astray." A light bulb may look *somewhat* brighter when we attend to it, but we have little trouble "inferring" how bright it actually is. As we shift our attentional focus around, we *know* that a light bulb's actual brightness doesn't change. Little cognitive effort seems to be required as we make such automatic "inferences." For this to happen, some compensatory mechanism likely operates as part of the perceptual process itself. So, if anything, this may be yet another argument in favor of the plausibility of inflation.

Earlier I mentioned that in Sperling post-cue settings, the impression of rich perception of all 12 letters is far from universal (Cova, Gaillard, and Kammerer 2020). When asked about it systematically, the majority of subjects did not report the impression of richness. But given that post-cue likely dampens uncued representations (Sergent et al. 2011), this may be just as expected. In a similar fashion as to how we should understand Carrasco's experiments, when the perceptual signal is enhanced, naturally we may expect the subjective appearance to be stronger. It may be the subtlety of the effect on appearance that really calls for an explanation. Likewise, for the 12 letters, we know that visual signals can't be equally strong for the post-cued and uncued letters. In this context, that some subjects reported some degree of uniform richness is rather remarkable. Inflation may help to account for that.

But just *how* does this compensatory mechanism work? How exactly do we inflate representations without detail, *as if* they are full of details? How do we go from confidence and decision mechanisms to apparent richness? We will explore these questions further in the rest of the chapter. We may not have the full answers just yet. But we will come back to these questions again in Chapter 7.

4.11 Filling-in?

Although the mechanisms for inflation aren't fully fleshed out, one commitment of the account is clear: apparent richness is not supported by actual detailed sensory content. This is in contrast with another popular account: "filling-in," which suggests that the details missing from the input stage are visually reconstructed internally. Typically, filling-in accounts involve having the details reconstructed at the early sensory level via top-down influence. If that's right, perhaps a local view can account for the apparent richness of experience too. That is, the higher areas may be involved, but only as distal causes. Ultimately, the constitutive mechanisms may be all within the early visual areas.

Vision scientists often favor this filling-in account. But that may be in part because of the problem of convenience, as mentioned in the Chapter 3: it is easier to *measure* such effects in the visual cortex.

One classic phenomenon of filling-in concerns the blind spot, that is, the part of the retinal location where the optic nerve bundle is, for which we lack sensitivity early on. We are typically not aware of the blind spot because the visual content is "filled-in," at the stage of the early visual cortex (Tong and Engel 2001). However, interestingly, even in this classic case of filling-in, inflation-like mechanisms may take place as well. It has been reported that filled-in content in the blind spot leads to higher subjective confidence, even though the content is no more reliable (Ehinger et al. 2017).

But there are also cases where the filling-in account does not seem to work well. The uniformity illusion is a powerful demonstration that a certain textural character of the central region of an image tends to be subjectively extrapolated into the periphery (Otten et al. 2017).

When one sees the illusion (Figure 4.3), does neural activity in the peripheral region of the early visual area misrepresent the central visual pattern? That would be the prediction of the filling-in account. Suárez-Pinilla et al. tested this indirectly using the psychophysics method of adaptation (2018). Recall from Section 2.10, where we discussed this method. The rationale is that usually when we look at a pattern for a long time, an ambiguous stimulus presented at the same location is more likely to look like the opposite of that pattern immediately afterwards, rather than the pattern itself. Sometimes we

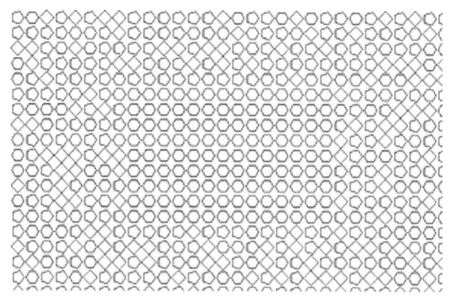

Figure 4.3 A demonstration of the uniformity illusion (taken from Otten et al. 2017); as
one stares at the center of the figure, over time, the entire pattern may look uniform,
even though when inspected carefully, the patterns in the periphery are varied

Reproduced from Otten, M., Pinto, Y., Paffen, C. L., Seth, A. K., & Kanai, R. (2017). The uniformity
illusion: Central stimuli can determine peripheral perception. *Psychological Science*, 28(1), 56-68. https://
doi.org/10.1177/0956797616672270

say that the representation for the pattern is *adapted out*, or that there is a
"repulsion" effect. The adapted pattern becomes less likely to win in a perceptual competition, when two alternative percepts are similarly plausible. This
is supposed to take place in the early visual cortex when a physical stimulus is
presented as the adaptor.

Suárez-Pinilla et al. applied this logic in a behavioral study (2018) to find
out the mechanisms for the uniformity illusion. They tested if the extrapolated
pattern in the periphery would have equal status to a physically presented
stimulus, in terms of its adaptation effects. The answer was no; the physical
pattern, not the illusory pattern, drove adaptation. The authors interpreted
this to mean that the illusion must take place in later areas, beyond the primary visual cortex.

There may be doubts about this claim because it is possible that the representations in the primary visual cortex were indeed changed under the illusion, just that the changes weren't in ways akin to actual presentation by
a physical stimulus. However, other studies of filling-in, such as those concerning the blind spot, typically find adaptation effects (Murakami 1995).
And yet they were absent here. So at least, we can say the mechanism for the
uniformity illusion is not identical to other filling-in effects.

Incidentally, under the uniformity illusion, the "extrapolated" patterns in the periphery also don't look *exactly* like physically presented patterns congruent with the center. This point was not emphasized in the original report, but is evident in the psychophysical data presented (Otten et al. 2017). When asked, subjects could distinguish the illusory extrapolation from an actually uniform image, much better than chance. One possibility is that the illusion is not "strong" enough to mimic the percept driven by physical stimuli. But phenomenologically, it is hard to deny that the illusion is powerful. So perhaps the mechanism isn't one of simple filling-in at the early sensory level. Something does differ at that level, allowing subjects to distinguish the illusory from the physically uniform scenarios, when needed. The illusory sense of uniformity probably arises at some *later stage* (Knotts, Michel, and Odegaard 2020).

4.12 Single Versus Multiple Levels of Representations

It should be clear that the above discussion isn't meant to be a rejection of the filling-in account in general. Filling-in certainly happens in many cases. But the point is that it is unlikely to account for all of the scenarios we've reviewed in this chapter: the speckled hen, Sperling's letter arrays and the uniformity illusion, for example. Multiple mechanisms are needed to account for the phenomenology of the unattended periphery.

Early on, Dennett wrote about the fallacy in thinking that consciousness must happen at a single place in the brain (1991). Unfortunately, this hasn't stopped researchers from debating whether subjective experience is determined by content in one specific brain area *or* another, as if these possibilities are necessarily mutually exclusive.

To illustrate the point, let us remind ourselves that we routinely make eye movements (i.e., saccades) up to a few times a second. And yet, the world looks relatively stable. Does it mean that eye movements have no impact on our visual phenomenology? That seems highly improbable. As you shift your gaze from one object to another, your retinal input changes. Certainly, we can feel a drastic difference if we think about it as we make these eye movements. But what if you don't think about those eye movements you make a few times a second, just as you normally don't—how does it feel? It is difficult to do the phenomenology justice, but it is probably fair to say that it makes sense these eye movements change your visual phenomenology drastically, and yet, *at the same time*, there is *also* another sense in which they don't.

Likewise, under the uniformity illusion, there is this similarly ambivalent sense that at once the periphery looks like it is an extrapolation from the center, *as if* the whole image is physically uniform; but at the same time, there is also a sense that it isn't identical to a physically uniform image.

Just for another example: when you look at a coin that is tilted sideways so it isn't facing you squarely. Does the coin look round or elliptical? There is a sense that you see the coin *as* round, precisely *because* you see it as elliptical (Noë 2004). Based on a series of ingenious experiments, Jorge Morales and colleagues concluded that our visual system simultaneously represents both (Morales, Bax, and Firestone 2020).

Dennett likened these situations to an author's being in the middle of writing a book (1991). One may be working on "multiple drafts," and they are all relevant. None alone is going to be the final word. So the analogy is that for our subjective visual experience, multiple representations at different parts of the visual cortex may all contribute. Sometimes, the instantaneous content does not have to be strictly coherent. If that's right, it may be rather silly to write off other researchers' favorite brain areas in favor of your own. They may all be just as important, as they contribute in different ways.

Importantly, from Chapters 2 and 3, we have argued that visual consciousness involves more than just the visual cortex. In the prefrontal cortex, representations are complex. Neurons don't just signal the presence and features of some external stimuli. To continue with the analogy, the prefrontal cortex may not just hold "drafts" of images representing the external world. There may also be "*post-it*" *notes*, labeling some *other* drafts as so-and-so, recommending appropriate further actions, just like what you'll find on the editor's desk: *This representation in MT (middle temporal area) is rich in detail. It has real potential. We should count on it with all our confidence.* Or: *This V1 representation looks terrible. Desk reject!*

This may be how the metacognitive mechanisms in the prefrontal cortex are relevant to the subjective experience of seeing—a point we will return to in Chapter 7. And if that's right, the global view isn't quite correct. The role of the prefrontal cortex is not to broadcast, amplify, ignite, or merely represent the content of consciousness. It acts more like an interpreter or a commentator—an idea that is of historical significance in the neuropsychology of consciousness (LeDoux, Michel, and Lau 2020).

4.13 A "Possible" Localist Rejoinder?

There is a position that I anticipate some die-hard localists may take. They may argue that much of the evidence reviewed here concerns high-level recognized and conceptualized details (e.g., letters, objects, and a person in a gorilla suit). Such details may well not be consciously perceived without attention. But some low-level, simple features like color and contrast may be uniformly represented across the visual field, giving us the "raw" phenomenology that can be stably rich (Haun 2020), independently from cognitive access and attention.

One problem with this view is, as we have already mentioned, some details like color and spatial resolution are actually known to be missing early on (e.g., from the retinal level). An interesting rejoinder from the localists may be to say that lack of details should not imply lack of subjective richness. We may just not be aware of what we do not represent (Anstis 1998). So perhaps we should not expect an active sense of blurriness or lack of color when the brain just does not keep track of the relevant information. That may be why we see the visual field as relatively uniform, despite the paucity of detailed information in the periphery.

But I am acutely aware that I do not see through the back of my head. I am not at all surprised by my lack of color vision there. This seems rather unlike the situation of peripheral vision, in which our behavioral deficits are often so surprising (Cohen, Botch, and Robertson 2020).

Let us suppose there is indeed this hypothetical level of representation characterizing the richness of phenomenology (Haun 2020). Just how does it relate to actual perception? We know that crowding applies to simple shapes and line segments, not just letters and other high level stimuli (Pelli and Tillman 2008). So for this account of uniform richness to work, it has to happen at some putative stage *prior* to crowding (Haun 2020). But crowding likely occurs as early as in V1 (Levi 2008). Meanwhile, as we discussed, attention is known to modulate activity as early as V1 as well (Sergent et al. 2011). In fact it could happen earlier still, in subcortical areas like the lateral geniculate nucleus (O'Connor et al. 2002; McAlonan, Cavanaugh, and Wurtz 2008). So where exactly are these simple representations supporting stable richness, resistant to both crowding and attentional modulation?

What I worry about is not only the lack of evidence at the moment. The problem is such putative representations are meant to be detached from actual perceptual *behavior*, which we know is constrained, for example, by crowding or attentional modulation. As such it is unclear how we can *ever* find any direct empirical evidence for them. In Chapter 6 we will discuss this problem further: that some localist claims are just unfalsifiable and empirically meaningless. The inflation account, on the other hand, can be supported by future discovery of concrete mechanisms in, for example, the prefrontal cortex.

4.14 Chapter Summary

In recent years, the debate on the richness of the phenomenology of perception has grown considerably. It is difficult to provide a comprehensive review of this literature. So here, I have not attempted to do so. Instead, I tried to give a gist of the landscape, to see where things stand on a coarser scale.

The debate is difficult, in large part because we cannot objectively and directly measure subjective experience. The problem is harder still for unattended experience, as self-reports can become dicey. So one may be tempted to say, to the extent that a percept isn't reported as such, we do not need to consider it truly conscious (Dehaene et al. 2006). That would make the life of a global theorist easier. But I find this view too restrictive. Certainly, there seem to be things that we consciously see but are so fleeting and complex that we may not be able to report about them. What we see seems not quite like just a gist or a simple statistical summary.

This impression of richness is often thought to be in favor of the local view. But the early sensory activity doesn't really seem to match the actually reported level of richness either (Cova, Gaillard, and Kammerer 2020). Some intuitions turn out to depend on data that aren't quite right.

Additionally, there is the problem of the relative *stability* of richness. However rich one thinks peripheral perception is, it just doesn't seem to be modulated so dramatically by the task that we are doing. Based on Lavie's load theory (2005), such changes in the tasks can be subtle. The tasks can be about the very same spatial location and stimuli and location, e.g. detecting a single feature versus conjunction of features. With such relatively small differences in the tasks, phenomenology for the peripheral background does not seem to change very much. And yet early sensory activities are reliably modulated (Schwartz et al. 2005).

So I introduced the concept of inflation and suggest that it may partly depend on mechanisms in the prefrontal cortex. This is congruent with what we've already discussed in Chapters 2 and 3: that the prefrontal cortex is constitutively involved in consciousness *somehow*. If that's correct, neither the global nor the local views are right on this matter. The phenomenology of perception may seem rich, but much of it may be internally "made up." Or we say it is "inflated," in the sense that the details aren't necessarily filled-in back at the level of early sensory representations. So perhaps the so-called raw feels aren't so raw after all. They hinge on sophisticated metacognitive and decisional processes, through which inflation occurs.

The true aficionados of raw feels may want them less "processed." They may demand raw feels that are truly untouched by cognition. But are there really such things? How would we ever know if they resemble how we feel at all? If we cut a piece of the early visual cortex out, put it on a petri-dish, and keep it alive, would the activity there reflect some raw experience, unbeknownst to anyone? Some authors have in fact urged us to consider such possibilities (as we will discuss in Chapters 6 and 9). But the present science suggests that there may be no need to go this far just yet. If the account of inflation works, we may already have what we need to account for the currently available data.

References

Abid G. Deflating inflation: The connection (or lack thereof) between decisional and metacognitive processes and visual phenomenology. *Neurosci Conscious* 2019;**2019**:niz015.

Alvarez GA. Representing multiple objects as an ensemble enhances visual cognition. *Trends Cogn Sci* 2011;**15**:122–131.

Anstis S. Picturing peripheral acuity. *Perception* 1998;**27**:817–825.

Beck J, Schneider KA. Attention and mental primer. *Mind Lang* 2017;**32**:463–494.

Block N. Consciousness, accessibility, and the mesh between psychology and neuroscience. *Behav Brain Sci* 2007;**30**:481–499; discussion 499–548.

Block N. Empirical science meets higher-order views of consciousness: Reply to Hakwan Lau and Richard Brown. In: A Pautz, D Stoljar (eds), *Blockheads! Essays on Ned Block's Philosophy of Mind and Consciousness*. MIT Press, 2019, 199–214.

Carandini M, Heeger DJ. Normalization as a canonical neural computation. *Nat Rev Neurosci* 2011;**13**:51–62.

Carrasco M. Visual attention: the past 25 years. *Vision Res* 2011;**51**:1484–1525.

Chabris C, Simons D. *The Invisible Gorilla: And Other Ways Our Intuitions Deceive Us*. Harmony, 2010.

Chisholm R. IV.—Discussions: The problem of the speckled hen. *Mind* 1942;**LI**:368–373.

Cohen MA, Botch TL, Robertson CE. The limits of color awareness during active, real-world vision. *Proc Natl Acad Sci U S A* 2020. https://doi.org/10.1073/pnas.1922294117.

Cohen MA, Dennett DC, Kanwisher N. What is the bandwidth of perceptual experience? *Trends Cogn Sci* 2016;**20**:324–335.

Cova F, Gaillard M, Kammerer F. Is the phenomenological overflow argument really supported by subjective reports? *Mind Lang* 2020;**36**(3):422–450. https://doi.org/10.1111/mila.12291.

Cowan N. The magic number 4 in short-term memory: A reconsideration of mental storage capacity. *The Behavioral and Brain Sciences*. 2001;**24**:87–114. doi: 10.1017/S0140525X01003922

Dehaene S, Changeux J-P, Naccache L et al. Conscious, preconscious, and subliminal processing: A testable taxonomy. *Trends Cogn Sci* 2006;**10**:204–211.

Dennett DC. *Consciousness Explained*. Little Brown, 1991.

Driver J. A selective review of selective attention research from the past century. *Br J Psychol* 2001;**92**(Part 1):53–78.

Ehinger BV, Häusser K, Ossandón JP et al. Humans treat unreliable filled-in percepts as more real than veridical ones. *Elife* 2017;**6**:e21761. https://doi.org/10.7554/eLife.21761.

de Gardelle V, Sackur J, Kouider S. Perceptual illusions in brief visual presentations. *Conscious Cogn* 2009;**18**:569–577.

Grove PM, Ashton J, Kawachi Y et al. Auditory transients do not affect visual sensitivity in discriminating between objective streaming and bouncing events. *J Vis* 2012;**12**:5.

Haun A. What is visible across the visual field? 2020;**1**:niab006. https://doi.org/10.1093/nc/niab006.

He S, Cavanagh P, Intriligator J. Attentional resolution and the locus of visual awareness. *Nature* 1996;**383**:334–337.

James W. *The Principles of Psychology*. Henry Holt and Company, 1910. https://doi.org/10.5962/bhl.title.47583.

King J-R, Dehaene S. A model of subjective report and objective discrimination as categorical decisions in a vast representational space. *Philos Trans R Soc Lond B Biol Sci* 2014;**369**:20130204.

Knotts JD, Michel M, Odegaard B. Defending subjective inflation: an inference to the best explanation. *Neurosci Conscious* 2020;**2020**:niaa025.

Knotts JD, Odegaard B, Lau H et al. Subjective inflation: Phenomenology's get-rich-quick scheme. *Curr Opin Psychol* 2019;**29**:49–55.

Kouider S, de Gardelle V, Dupoux E. Partial awareness and the illusion of phenomenal consciousness. *Behavioral and Brain Sciences* 2007;**30**:510–511.

Landman R, Spekreijse H, Lamme VAF. Large capacity storage of integrated objects before change blindness. *Vision Res* 2003;**43**:149–164.

Lavie N. Distracted and confused?: Selective attention under load. *Trends Cogn Sci* 2005;**9**:75–82.

LeDoux JE, Michel M, Lau H. A little history goes a long way toward understanding why we study consciousness the way we do today. *Proceedings of the National Academy of Sciences* 2020;**117**:6976–6984.

Levi DM. Crowding--an essential bottleneck for object recognition: A mini-review. *Vision Res* 2008;**48**:635–654.

Levin DT, Angelone BL. The visual metacognition questionnaire: a measure of intuitions about vision. *Am J Psychol* 2008;**121**:451–472.

Li FF, VanRullen R, Koch C et al. Rapid natural scene categorization in the near absence of attention. *Proc Natl Acad Sci U S A* 2002;**99**:9596–9601.

Li MK, Lau H, Odegaard B. An investigation of detection biases in the unattended periphery during simulated driving. *Atten Percept Psychophys* 2018;**80**:1325–1332.

McAlonan K, Cavanaugh J, Wurtz RH. Guarding the gateway to cortex with attention in visual thalamus. *Nature* 2008;**456**:391–394.

Meyerhoff HS, Scholl BJ. Auditory-induced bouncing is a perceptual (rather than a cognitive) phenomenon: Evidence from illusory crescents. *Cognition* 2018;**170**:88–94.

Michel M. Consciousness science underdetermined: A short history of endless debates. *Ergo* 2019;**6**. https://doi.org/10.3998/ergo.12405314.0006.028.

Michel M, Lau H. Is blindsight possible under signal detection theory? Comment on Phillips (2021). *Psychol Rev* 2021;**128**:585–591.

Morales J, Bax A, Firestone C. Sustained representation of perspectival shape. *Proc Natl Acad Sci U S A* 2020;117;**26**:14873–14882https://doi.org/10.1073/pnas.2000715117.

Murakami I. Motion aftereffect after monocular adaptation to filled-in motion at the blind spot. *Vision Res* 1995;**35**:1041–5.

Neisser U, Becklen R. Selective looking: Attending to visually specified events. *Cognitive Psychology* 1975;**7**:480–494.

Noë A. *Action in Perception*. MIT Press, 2004.

O'Connor DH, Fukui MM, Pinsk MA et al. Attention modulates responses in the human lateral geniculate nucleus. *Nat Neurosci* 2002;**5**:1203–1209.

Odegaard B, Chang MY, Lau H et al. Inflation versus filling-in: why we feel we see more than we actually do in peripheral vision. *Phil Trans Royal Society B* 2018;**373**:20170345 https://doi.org/10.1101/263244.

Otten M, Pinto Y, Paffen CLE et al. The uniformity illusion. *Psychol Sci* 2017;**28**:56–68.

Pelli DG, Tillman KA. The uncrowded window of object recognition. *Nat Neurosci* 2008;**11**:1129–1135.

Peters MAK, Ro T, Lau H. Who's afraid of response bias? *Neuroscience of Consciousness* 2016;**2016**:niw001.

Polat U, Sagi D. The relationship between the subjective and objective aspects of visual filling-in. *Vision Res* 2007;**47**:2473–2481.

Rahnev D, Maniscalco B, Graves T et al. Attention induces conservative subjective biases in visual perception. *Nature Neuroscience* 2011;**14**:1513–1515.

Rosenholtz R. Demystifying visual awareness: Peripheral encoding plus limited decision complexity resolve the paradox of rich visual experience and curious perceptual failures. *Atten Percept Psychophys* 2020;**82**:901–925 https://doi.org/10.3758/s13414-019-01968-1.

Schwartz S, Vuilleumier P, Hutton C et al. Attentional load and sensory competition in human vision: Modulation of fMRI responses by load at fixation during task-irrelevant stimulation in the peripheral visual field. *Cereb Cortex* 2005;**15**:770–786.

Sergent C, Ruff CC, Barbot A et al. Top–down modulation of human early visual cortex after stimulus offset supports successful postcued report. *Journal of Cognitive Neuroscience* 2011;**23**:1921–1934.

Sligte IG, Vandenbroucke ARE, Scholte HS et al. Detailed sensory memory, sloppy working memory. *Front Psychol* 2010;**1**:175.

Solovey G, Graney GG, Lau H. A decisional account of subjective inflation of visual perception at the periphery. *Atten Percept Psychophys* 2015;**77**:258–271.

Sperling G. The information available in brief visual presentations. *Psychological Monographs: General and Applied* 1960;**74**:1–29.

Suárez-Pinilla M, Seth AK, Roseboom W. The illusion of uniformity does not depend on the primary visual cortex: Evidence from sensory adaptation. *i-Perception* 2018;**9**:204166951880050.

Tong F, Engel SA. Interocular rivalry revealed in the human cortical blind-spot representation. *Nature* 2001;**411**:195–199.

Toscani M, Mamassian P, Valsecchi M. Underconfidence in peripheral vision. *J Vis* 2021;**21**:2.

Treue S. Neural correlates of attention in primate visual cortex. *Trends in Neurosciences* 2001;**24**:295–300.

Tyler CW. Peripheral color demo. *Iperception* 2015;**6**:2041669515613671.

Valsecchi M, Koenderink J, van Doorn A et al. Prediction shapes peripheral appearance. *J Vis* 2018;**18**:21.

Witt JK, Taylor JET, Sugovic M et al. Signal detection measures cannot distinguish perceptual biases from response biases. *Perception* 2015;**44**:289–300.

Zizlsperger L, Sauvigny T, Haarmeier T. Selective attention increases choice certainty in human decision making. *PLOS One* 2012;**7**:e41136.

5

What Good Is Consciousness?

5.1 Evolution

Most of us agree that consciousness emerged at some time through our evolutionary history. Many also find probable that it is a relatively recent invention; simple organisms like bacteria are presumably not conscious. But how about insects, fish, birds, rodents, and the like? We will address this question more fully in Chapter 7.

The point here is: even if we accept this evolutionary outlook, it does not mean that consciousness is selected *because* it provides unique functional advantages for our survival—not necessarily.

That's because evolution is a long and complex process. Take a "uniquely human" feature as an example: having chins, that structure sticking out by the edge of our lower jaw. Other mammals do not have it, not even the nonhuman primates. Is it because it allows us to speak? Or is it to protect our relatively fragile throats in melee combats? Or maybe it has something to do with bipedalism—maybe human toddlers fall on their faces so often that they need a bony jaw structure to protect them from damage? It may be amusing to try to come up with stories like these. But there is just no such simple answer (Holton et al. 2015).

Likewise, consciousness could also have evolved mostly as a byproduct (Robinson, Maley, and Piccinini 2015) or for reasons that we do not intuitively expect. Like others, I too find it hard to believe that it really has no function whatsoever. But the point is not that there's decidedly no function. The point is that the answer may not be so obvious from the outset. Beyond "just so" stories, we need direct empirical evidence. Unfortunately, as I will explain, so far most of the evidence we have isn't very strong.

5.2 Libet & Volition

Benjamin Libet is often credited for having challenged the existence of free will from a neurophysiological perspective (Libet et al. 1983). But his famous study

In Consciousness We Trust. Hakwan Lau, Oxford University Press. © Hakwan Lau 2022.
DOI: 10.1093/oso/9780198856771.003.0006

was in part based on an older finding: Kornhuber and Deecke (1965) showed that there was electrophysiological activity preceding simple spontaneous movements. This activity, called the *readiness potential*, was measured by averaging electroencephalograms recorded from the scalp. What was surprising was that this activity can start as early as a whole second before the movement.

Libet reasoned that the early onset may be due to the lack of complete spontaneity on the subjects' parts. But even after discarding blocks of trials in which they reported any recollection of inadvertent "preplanning," the readiness potential was still detectable at up to about half a second prior to movement. That seemed odd: for a truly spontaneous act, it doesn't seem to require that much time to prepare. Confirming this, Libet and colleagues showed that people only reported consciously initiating the movement about a quarter of a second before actual execution. So the brain seems to start nonconsciously initiating the action prior to that.

Perhaps it isn't so bad that our conscious intentions aren't the "first unmoved movers." We should accept that maybe our actions aren't so truly *de novo*. Although they may seem spontaneous to our conscious selves, they may have nonconscious origins too. But if consciousness arises some time before movement execution, perhaps it means we can consciously edit our actions before it's too late. Possibly, we are still a part of the causal chain.

But of course, this would not be possible if the action was already fully determined and predictable at the early stage of nonconscious initiation, before we become consciously aware of the intention. In that case, by the time our conscious intention arises, it would be too late. In the literature, sometimes the words *determined* and *predicted* were used in this context, giving this impression (e.g. Soon et al. 2008). But in fact, the nature of the action at those early nonconscious stages can only be very weakly predicted statistically. So perhaps the conscious intention that arises later can still play a major causal role.

Others wonder if the early nonconscious reflects anything specific to the action at all. Perhaps it is just some general "noise" in the brain. But single cell physiological studies in monkeys have shown that this is unlikely (Romo and Schultz 1987). Prior to spontaneous actions, some neurons within the motor systems fire up to over 2 seconds before the movement onset. These neurons code specific properties of the movements.

So, instead of being driven by nonspecific motor "noise," the readiness potential probably reflects the fluctuation of specific preparatory activity, to be detected consciously when it passes a certain threshold (Nikolov, Rahnev, and Lau 2010; Schurger, Sitt, and Dehaene 2012). This may allow some half-formed, and yet specific, motor plans to reach our awareness, for potential "editing" prior to action execution.

5.3 Free Will as an Illusion

As such, the question seems open regarding whether our conscious intentions play a causal role. When I was a PhD student in Dick Passingham's lab, I set out to test this question. Using functional magnetic resonance imaging (fMRI), we first localized where the representations of conscious intention may be. Like the direct brain stimulation patient study mentioned in Section 3.10 (Fried et al. 1991), we linked intention to a medial prefrontal area called the presupplementary motor area (Lau et al. 2004; Lau, Rogers, and Passingham 2006). This also is roughly the same area from which they recorded single cell activities in the study in monkeys mentioned in Section 5.3 (Romo and Schultz 1987), or just slightly anterior to that. I then used transcranial magnetic stimulation (TMS) to stimulate the area, and found that people's retrospective reports of the onset of intention could actually be modulated even *after* the action was completed (Lau, Rogers, and Passingham 2007). We did control studies to rule out that this finding was just a general memory effect; it was specific to the time around action completion. The effect was also specific to the reported onset of intention, but not to the movement itself, nor the reported onset of other events, like tactile sensations.

After stimulation, subjects reported their intention to have started earlier— as if TMS injected some extra activity into the brain area, which was mistaken as a meaningful intention signal. So, overall they thought they had been intending to make the movement for longer, compared to when their brains were not being stimulated. Importantly, if this interpretation was true, it means that the mechanisms giving rise to consciousness must not be very precise in tracking the intention signal "online." Instead, as the late Daniel Wegner suggested, perhaps it is all loosely reconstructed after the fact. The so-called conscious will may very well be an illusion (2004).

These studies probably set me on a good path of inquiry. I still think the results are more or less correct. Our sense of volitional agency may indeed depend on late-stage cognitive processing, at least in part. That is to say, it is unlikely a direct instant readout of our internal motoric signals, just as the TMS findings suggest. We will revisit this issue in Section 8.5.

But I describe these studies relatively briefly here, because by the time I finished my PhD, I had become frustrated by these experiments. It is a very odd thing to ask people to make these "spontaneous" movements "at any time they like," and to report the onset of "intention" afterwards. If consciousness is to serve some important survival functions, I doubt it concerns primarily situations of this sort.

5.4 Impossible Situation

When I was in grad school, Dehaene's global view had already started to dominate. In particular I remember reading a wonderful piece by Naccache and Dehaene (2001), in which they spelled out some predictions of their theory. It was so clearly written and intellectually honest that it set a standard for all of us to follow.

One prediction was based on the finding that once the subjects understood certain task instructions, they could apply this "task set" to subliminal stimuli. By "task set" we mean the rules of the task, in terms of what sensory stimuli require what motor responses. For example, the task may be to decide if a number was bigger or smaller than five, and to press keys with different hands accordingly. Once they started doing the task, motor activity for the correct hand response could be triggered by visually masked numbers that were invisible. The interpretation is that once the task set was established, information could meaningfully go from a perceptual process to the motor mechanisms, all without consciousness. We call this a "priming" effect: a subliminal stimulus can induce some level of preparedness for the relevant representations. So once a task set was on, a subliminal stimulus can "prime" the relevant motor response.

However, based on the global workspace theory, they predicted that the establishment of the task set itself should require consciousness. That is because the very function of the global workspace is to exert top-down control to coordinate how the perceptual and motor modules are linked. They famously called it an "Impossible Situation" for subliminal stimuli to influence this initial process of setting up the task set (Naccache and Dehaene 2001).

Being a contrarian (and deluded too, as I mentioned in Section 2.11), I set out to challenge that prediction. I reasoned that, in a sense, what they found was that in a single case, a simple function (motor priming by invisible stimuli) could be exercised without consciousness. From there, it is natural to think that consciousness may be required for a more complex function (the establishment of a task set based on instruction). But did they try hard enough to see if the more complex function really couldn't also be exercised nonconsciously? Maybe with a stronger nonconscious signal, it could?

So, the first project I did as a postdoc was to test this (Lau and Passingham 2007). In the experiment we presented a figure to tell the subjects if they needed to do a phonological or semantic task on that trial. In the phonological task they had to judge if a word was disyllabic. In the semantic task they had to judge if the word referred to a concrete object. Because they saw the instruction figure before the word appeared, during the time between the two they had an opportunity to establish the "task set" quickly. Interestingly, we found that a subliminal instruction figure could also influence task set establishment. Let's say they were presented with a highly visible instruction figure telling them to prepare for a phonological task. When we inserted an invisible figure telling them to prepare for a semantic task before the visible instruction figure providing different instructions, this created a kind of nonconscious conflict. Overall, subjects would still be mostly doing the phonological task as consciously instructed, but they were slower and less accurate—as if they were nonconsciously distracted to do the other task as well. Using fMRI, we showed that when they were "primed" this way, there was less phonological-related activity, and more semantically related activity, in the relevant brain regions. The nonconscious conflicts also led to more activity in areas of the prefrontal cortext, which typically responds to cognitive and response conflicts.

5.5 More "Impossible" Cases

After I moved to Columbia University, my then graduate student Doby Rahnev took this one step further. He presented the subliminal task instruction stimuli outside of attentional focus. And yet, the task set seems to be successfully primed nonconsciously in the same way (Rahnev, Huang, and Lau 2012).

Simon van Gaal has also done similar studies (van Gaal et al. 2008, 2010, 2011; van Gaal, Lamme, and Ridderinkhof 2010). Together with colleagues holding the local view, he mostly focused on response inhibition, another task that is linked to prefrontal higher cognitive functions. So, in these tasks subjects had to make a response quickly. On some trials, there might be a "no-go" or "stop" signal, so they had to withhold the prepared response. They found that a subliminal "no-go" signal could slow down prepared responses too, as if some degree of inhibition took place. It also led to more prefrontal activity, typically reflecting inhibitory control in these settings.

Meanwhile, Dehaene's own lab has also reported various cases in which nonconscious stimuli can influence higher cognitive functions like error detection (Charles et al. 2013; Charles, King and Dehaene 2014) and working memory (King, Pescetelli, and Dehaene 2016; Trübutschek et al. 2017, 2019; Trübutschek, Marti, and Dehaene 2019). As I will explain in Section 5.6, there may be some concerns as to whether these stimuli were truly invisible. Also, in the case of "working" memory, perhaps these are really only cases of brief sensory memory; one may not be able to actively manipulate the memory content, to protect it against distractors, for example. But all the same, it is remarkable that a strong proponent of the global view himself accepts these cases as showing that nonconscious stimuli can influence such high-level processes.

Together with other colleagues, Ryan Scott and Zoltan Dienes also did some studies showing that nonconscious stimuli likely can go through some central mechanisms (Scott et al. 2018). Again using a priming approach, they showed that nonconscious stimuli from one sensory modality (e.g., hearing) can influence processing in another modality (e.g., vision). For this to work, presumably the nonconscious information has to go through some central mechanisms that link up processes from the different modalities. But if such central mechanisms are what make information conscious, that seems … just impossible.

So, taking together all of the evidence discussed, the "impossible situation" as predicted by Naccache and Dehaene (2001) doesn't seem so impossible after all. I felt smug for a while, as I thought we had falsified the global view. But later I came to think these studies may not really tell us that much.

5.6 The Limits of Subliminal Priming Experiments

We can all agree that the primary function of having legs is for locomotion. It allows us to move around. Lower limbs are probably selected through evolution because of this useful function. But if we remove the legs of a small insect, it may still be able to wiggle around a little. Or maybe it has wings too, so it can fly around.

By analogy, consciousness may also have the primary functions of higher cognitive control, including establishing task sets and response inhibition. Without consciousness, we can exercise these functions *a little bit*, and this is perhaps all that the priming studies showed. Perhaps it is only with consciousness that we can drive these functions fully. So consciousness may be selected through evolution for this reason after all.

This is somewhat related to our tendency to think in terms of necessity. As I have argued in Sections 2.3, 3.2, and 4.3, this is often misguided. In studying the functions of consciousness, we often want to show that it is "necessary" for certain functions, but not others. But it does not work this way. There are several problems.

The first is logical. Consciousness may not be strictly necessary for a function to be exercised to some minimal extent. But it could be necessary for the function to be exercised *more effectively*. Or maybe there are multiple ways to exercise these functions, and consciousness is one of the more obvious and economical ways, conveniently picked out by evolution. In this sense, testing for necessity just doesn't directly answer our question.

Nor is it very practical. Like attention and many other psychological constructs, consciousness isn't something we can neatly turn on and off. When we apply visual masking, how do we know it is effective? We typically make subjects do forced-choice detection or discrimination tasks to ascertain that they are at chance, meaning no perception occurs. But to statistically prove that something is completely absent is difficult. With very many trials, even very weak stimuli may be detectable or discriminable above chance. Showing a nonsignificant result is easy; one only needs to test it with an insufficient number of trials, or to measure things poorly. But proving that something truly is at chance is a statistical challenge. So, this is the second problem: convincing demonstration of subliminality.

In recent years, some authors have given up on showing that these stimuli are truly invisible in the sense of completely lacking detectability or discriminability. Instead, they took subjective reports of the lack of awareness at face value. Using these methods, various authors have claimed to have found evidence for nonconscious working memory (King, Pescetelli, and Dehaene 2016; Trübutschek et al. 2017, 2019; Trübutschek, Marti, and Dehaene 2019), nonconscious metacognition (Charles et al. 2013; Charles, King, and Dehaene 2014; Jachs et al. 2015), and blindsight in normal observers (Hesselmann, Hebart, and Malach 2011).

I, too, have emphasized the importance of subjective reports. But in most of the studies I reviewed in the previous chapters, the usage was to compare different levels of reported awareness across conditions within the same subjects. The point was to show that the level of awareness differed between the conditions, not that one condition lacked awareness completely. By traditional psychophysics standards, it is not acceptable to infer the lack of awareness based on subjective reports alone (Macmillan and Douglas Creelman 2004). This is because subjects use these reports based on rather arbitrary criteria. If we give people the options "no awareness," "some awareness," and "high awareness," naturally they will say "no awareness" on some of the weakest trials. But this may only reflect that they understand these options in relative rather than absolute terms.

When Megan Peters was a postdoc in my lab at UCLA, she did studies to control for this "criterion" problem (Peters and Lau 2015). Instead of asking people to rate their visibility or awareness on some arbitrary scale, she asked them to compare two consecutive presentations. The logic is: If a stimulus was truly invisible, one should not be able to distinguish it from another stimulus lacking any useful information. If subjects were asked to bet on their ability to correctly identify one of them, they shouldn't know which one to bet. With this method, she has shown that at least for the case of blindsight in normal observers, it was likely to all due to criterion artifacts—at least for the kind stimuli typically used in previous studies (see also Knotts, Lau, and Peters 2018). That is, there was no convincing evidence for nonconscious perception in normal observers, when the possibility of criterion artifact was taken into account, using her criterion-free forced-choice betting method. So care must be taken before we take subjects' reported lack of awareness at face value.

There is a third problem with subliminal priming studies, which I think is just as troubling. In experiments, when we use, for instance, visual masking to render some stimuli invisible, we are also changing other things. The confounders introduced back in Chapter 2 apply. With the mask on, there is obviously a stimulus difference. A bigger problem, though, is the task-performance capacity confounder. If the invisible stimuli are just weak, then of course many functions will not be driven so well by them. But it may not be the lack of consciousness per se that matters. Perhaps we just haven't found a way to keep a nonconscious signal strong enough.

5.7 Performance Matching & Statistical Power

When I was at Columbia University, a postdoc in my lab, Ai Koizumi, did some work to address this last issue (Koizumi, Maniscalco, and Lau 2015). The idea was similar to the way we deal with task-performance capacity confounders in Chapter 2: she found a pair of stimuli in which task performance was directly matched, and yet they showed some difference in subjective visibility. In the study we actually measured confidence rather than visibility, but I believe that would have worked similarly. Ai-san showed that stimuli perceived to be subjectively stronger didn't really facilitate task set preparation (Koizumi, Maniscalco, and Lau 2015). There were some subtle effects on inhibition strategy, but overall inhibition was no more effective.

So I was back to thinking that maybe the global view was in some trouble after all. When performance capacity was controlled for, a sheer subjective difference in perception did not lead to functional advantages for these higher cognitive control functions. So consciousness probably wasn't as functionally important as the global view holds.

But I have to acknowledge, there was also a problem in our study (Koizumi, Maniscalco, and Lau 2015): statistical power was rather limited. This is a general issue with our way of addressing the performance-capacity confounders in subjects from the general population. It is very difficult to get a large effect on subjective perception while having task-performance capacity matched. As such, null results need to be interpreted with caution. Just because we did not find functional advantages there for consciousness doesn't mean there aren't such advantages. Maybe we just needed more subjects for a subtle effect to be detected.

Brian Maniscalco and others have recently spelled out a framework for how to design better studies of this sort, with adequate power (Maniscalco et al 2020). But we are yet to see more new studies done this way.

This issue of lack of statistical power is not specific to performance-matching studies. It applies whenever our expected effect sizes are small. Small effects aren't easily detected with a small sample. To verify that they are truly absent, rather than missed because they are so weak, we need a lot of data. So this is a problem for most of the subliminal priming studies too. When the stimuli are masked to become invisible, we can't really expect the effects to be very big. This can be yet another problem with subliminal priming.

With all these caveats in mind, next, I'll highlight a few findings that I think are relatively promising.

5.8 Inhibition & Exclusion

Earlier in Section 5.4, I mentioned that it may be possible to trigger response inhibition nonconsciously. Such findings have been taken by local theorists as challenges to the global view. However, it is possible that consciousness allows inhibition to work better.

Navindra Persaud and Alan Cowey have tested the blindsight patient GY (Persaud and Cowey 2008). GY is the same patient whom we already described in Chapter 2. Blindsight mostly affected GY's right visual field. Persaud and Cowey adopted a version of Jacoby's "exclusion" task (Jacoby, Jones, and Dolan 1998). They asked GY to report the opposite of what was shown. That is, he had to report "up" if the stimulus was actually presented in the lower quadrant, and vice versa. For stimuli presented in the "normal" field, this was easy to do. However, for the "blind" field, not only did GY have some difficulty doing this, curiously, he made more errors as the stimulus was shown at a higher contrast. Under the lack of awareness, the stimulus seemed to have driven his responses in an automatic fashion, leading to his failure to "exclude" or inhibit the natural and prepotent reaction.

This was only a single patient. But an elegant study from Takeo Watanabe's lab (Tsushima, Sasaki, and Watanabe 2006) also found something similar in an fMRI study with subjects from the general population. In that study the inhibition concerned some irrelevant, distractor stimuli presented in the background. The subjects were required to focus on a central task and to ignore these distractors. It was found that the distractor effect was actually the strongest when the stimuli were at an intermediate strength, around perceptual threshold. The interpretation is, when the distractors were weak, they didn't have much impact. But when they were strong and highly visible, subjects were able to actively inhibit their influence. Congruent with this interpretation, activity in the lateral prefrontal cortex was higher when the distractors were visible. It was as if some inhibitory functions there were only engaged when the distractors were consciously perceived.

These studies are intriguing because they showed that an increase in stimulus strength does not always lead to more effective inhibition. Perhaps inhibitory functions kick in only when consciousness is engaged. But in these studies, the nonconscious stimuli were weak. In Persaud and Cowey (2008), although the stimuli presented to the blindfield were physically as strong as those presented to the normal, sighted field, the associating performance capacity was not matched. To really address the issue of performance capacity confounder, future studies can test whether even very strong nonconscious signals would fail to trigger inhibition as effectively as weak conscious signals.

5.9 Metacognition

With other colleagues (including myself), Navindra Persaud also tested GY's metacognitive abilities between the "normal" and "blind" field (Persaud et al. 2011). Interestingly, GY was willing to bet money on his performance in the "blind" field as much as he was for the "normal" field. Presumably, it means he was "aware" of his good performance there, in a cognitive sense. But over trials, his bets did not track accuracy so well in the "blind" field, as compared to the "normal" field. He did bet higher on his correct trials over his incorrect trials, meaning he probably had some metacognitive ability even in the "blind" field. But this ability was higher in the "normal" field, even for weaker stimuli giving rise to lower task performance than in the "blind" field.

The idea that consciousness may facilitate metacognition is not new (Baars 1988; Shea and Frith 2019). What is intriguing is that, here we have a positive finding that does not suffer from the task-performance capacity confounders. As in inhibition, the function of metacognition was not completely abolished under the lack of consciousness. But consciousness seems to facilitate it even when task-performance capacity was matched (or when it was lower than in the nonconscious condition).

5.10 Endogenous Attention

Because inhibition and metacognition are functions associated with mechanisms in the prefrontal cortex, one may think that maybe the global view is not so challenged after all. That is, although priming studies showed that nonconscious stimuli can exercise some prefrontal functions (as reviewed in Sections 5.4 and 5.5), perhaps consciousness will always allow us to exercise these functions more effectively. Unfortunately, this is unlikely to be true for all prefrontal functions.

For a counter example, let us reconsider the relationship between attention and consciousness, which is complex, as we have reviewed already in Chapter 4. There, we were mostly concerned with how attention may modulate subjective experience. But one can also ask: For stimuli that are not consciously perceived, can they benefit from attentional cueing too? That is, if we attend to these nonconscious stimuli, do we speed up the processing as much as we do for consciously perceived stimuli? In particular, when an attentional cue is given symbolically , rather than physically around the stimulus in question, we say this is a form of endogenous attention. In this case, the subjects have to process the meaning of the cue, rather than to act reflexively. Endogenous cueing is believed to depend on prefrontal mechanisms.

Bob Kentridge and colleagues have tested this on patient GY (Kentridge, Heywood, and Weiskrantz 2004). They presented a visual cue in the center of the screen, where GY could see consciously, to indicate to the patient where the subsequent target stimulus was likely to appear. The target was a bar that was either horizontal or vertical, presented to GY's blindfield. Turns out, when the cue was predictive of the location of the target, it helped patient GY respond more quickly—by over 100 milliseconds. Because normal cueing effects for visible stimuli are generally not bigger than this, we can say that the stimulus presented to the blindfield didn't seem to suffer in this specific context, despite the lack of subjective awareness.

These authors have also found that this kind of cueing also works when the attentional cue was presented in the blindfield, such that GY did not see the cue stimulus. However, the effect in this kind of nonconscious cueing, in which the cue stimulus itself was not consciously perceived, seems to be smaller (Kentridge, Heywood, and Weiskrantz 1999). So it is possible that consciousness may play some role there. But others have also found fairly robust attentional cueing effects, in subjects from the general population, using stimuli rendered invisible (Zhang et al. 2012; Huang et al. 2020).

5.11 Intuitively "Improbable" Situations?

The examples discussed in Sections 5.7–5.10 hopefully help illustrate that assessing the functional advantages associated with consciousness is no trivial matter. We really have to go through the empirical specifics, in a case by case manner.

Why is it that some prefrontal functions seem to benefit from consciousness (i.e., having the relevant stimuli consciously perceived), while others don't? That's probably because the prefrontal cortex is a substantial part of the brain. Many different cognitive functions reside within this brain region. Let us suppose, for a moment, that some specific prefrontal mechanisms are key to consciousness, just like what global theories suggest. So when a stimulus fails to generate a conscious experience, it could be that the entire prefrontal cortex is compromised. Or it could be that just some specific mechanisms within the prefrontal cortex responsible for consciousness are compromised. Alternatively, it could be that all these mechanisms are intact, but the sensory signals somehow fail to reach the prefrontal cortex, because of some early sensory deficits. Because multiple mechanisms are likely involved in the entire chain of processes, without direct evidence it is hard to say what is definitely the problem when a perceptual process fails to lead to a subjective conscious experience.

In other words, it is also difficult to pinpoint what functions will *always* be compromised in nonconscious processing. A perceptual process can fail to be conscious in different ways (Block 2016). To get at this issue, we probably need a theoretical model outlining what really is the mechanism of consciousness. We probably need to understand how the different components interact to support subjective experience. But even then, when that mechanism breaks down, there may be "back-up" systems. Understanding this is complicated business.

Despite that, some of the evidence discussed is relatively informative. It is clear that not all prefrontal functions are enhanced by consciousness. But it seems that even when the performance confound is not an issue, as in blindsight, the lack of consciousness seems to impair metacognition.

What else is unlikely to be performed well by the blindsight patient? Without the relevant direct experimental data, if you allow me to speculate based on my own interaction with GY (Persaud and Lau 2008): I suspect it is generally impossible for any blindsight patient to spontaneously form the belief with certainty that a specific stimulus is presented. When forced, GY makes a guess. But the perceptual process never impinges on his rational decision-making system directly and spontaneously.

Also, although we never did this experiment, I suspect we could have: let's say we set up a forced-choice experiment, where we ask the patient to discriminate between horizontal versus vertical bars. If on some trials we present to him a 45-degree-tilted bar, very clearly, I suspect he would be none the wiser, and just proceeds to make his guess as to whether it is horizontal or vertical. He probably would not say: "Well this was not expected. What is this?" Or if we presented to him something he had never seen before, like a computer generated fractal image, he probably would not say: "I haven't seen anything like this before. Is there an error?"

But these are my guesses. I do not have empirical evidence for these claims. I spell them out here because, in a way, if GY behaved not as I hypothesized, I would actually doubt whether he genuinely lacked subjective experience in his blindfield. That is to say, this would be improbable on a *conceptual* level. There seems to be something intrinsic to what it takes for one to lack subjective experience. But this clearly is a theoretical matter, open to debate. We shall address these more properly in Chapters 7–9 (especially Sections 9.4–9.9).

5.12 DecNef & Threat Reduction

Why do we rely so much on single-patient studies in blindsight? The reason is as explained earlier in Section 5.6: These studies allow us to see what can be achieved with a nonconscious and yet strong internal signal. With masking, conscious visibility can be abolished, but the internal perceptual signal is also mostly gone. With such weak residual signals we are stuck with some small effects, such as those typically reported in subliminal priming studies. These effects are neither easy to interpret nor to replicate.

There is a way around this with subjects from the general population. The trick is to go directly into their brains and look for these nonconscious strong signals. My colleagues in Japan, Kazuhisa Shibata, Yuka Sasaki, Takeo Watanabe, and Mitsuo Kawato, have pioneered a technique called decoded neurofeedback, which we sometimes call DecNef for short (Shibata et al. 2011; Watanabe et al. 2018). The idea is that we can apply multivoxel pattern analysis (MVPA) to fMRI data online (i.e., in real-time). In Chapter 2 we already described this kind of analysis. Essentially, in MVPA we look for fine-grained patterns in fMRI data within a region, in order to extract meaningful content from them. This differs from the more traditional approaches, which tend to focus on the overall level of activity in an area.

Interestingly, people are generally unaware of the spontaneous fluctuations of these decoded internal brain signals. For example, we can present red lines and green lines to subjects. These stimuli will activate visual areas to similar overall degrees. But with MVPA, we can distinguish between trials in which red versus green lines are presented. When there is no color stimuli, these same decoded internal signals still fluctuate spontaneously. So, sometimes our brains look as if the line presented was mildly representing green or red. But, of course, we do not consciously "see" this kind of internal fluctuation. In fact, when we asked subjects to directly guess the content of their decoded internal signal, they were generally at chance (Shibata et al. 2011; Watanabe et al. 2018).

But do these decoded internal signals have any cognitive or behavioral impact on the subject? Turns out, they do, in fairly powerful ways. For example, Ai Koizumi did a study in which she paired these red- and green-line visual patterns with unpleasant electric shocks (Koizumi et al. 2016). After a while, subjects showed physiological reactions to these colored patterns alone, even without shock, as if they were physiologically threatened by the line patterns themselves. After that, we used DecNef to see if we could reduce this learned threat response. In one group of subjects, we paired these decoded signals representing red lines with reward, during fMRI. (In another group we targeted green-line patterns as a counter-balanced control.) During this period, no colored patterns were presented. But if the nonconscious decoded brain signal looked as if it was representing red, we gave feedback to the subjects to indicate that they earned some money (on the order of a few cents). This way, we hoped that the brain patterns previously associated with threat will now be "counter-conditioned" with reward. The subjects were blind to the purpose of the study; from their perspective, they just played hundreds of trials of this "mental slot machine," and earned some tens of dollars over a few days.

To our pleasant surprise, the hypothesis worked. After a few hours of DecNef, when presented with the red-line patterns, their physiological reactions were indeed diminished, as if the shock-paired stimuli became less threatening somehow. Importantly, this was specific to the brain signals which went through the feedback procedure. Subjects showed just as much physiological reactions to the green-line patterns, the decoded signals for which were not rewarded through DecNef.

This served as a promising proof-of-concept. Vincent Tascherau-Dumouchel, a postdoc in my lab at UCLA, thought we could take it one step further. Perhaps we can actually use this to reduce common phobia in people (Taschereau-Dumouchel et al. 2018). To do this we decoded voxel patterns for visual objects and animals, including the commonly feared ones like spiders and snakes. As in Koizumi et al., using DecNef, we paired the decoded internal brain signals with reward. Conceptually it replicated our earlier findings. Physiological-threat responses were reduced when subjects saw the images of the feared animals, specifically for the ones paired with reward only. Because the feedback and randomization procedures were all conducted by the computer, the entire process was double-blind placebo-controlled too.

5.13 Clinical Applications?

Can DecNef one day work in clinical settings for real? We do not know yet. As I'm writing, my lab is currently conducting a clinical trial co-led by my UCLA colleague Michelle Craske, who is an expert on anxiety disorders. One challenge is that to decode these voxel patterns, we typically show many images to the subjects while they are in the fMRI scanner. But for patients who are unable to tolerate seeing these images over and over again, they may as well go through conventional psychotherapy, which is arguably more economical. For phobia and posttraumatic stress disorders, traditional therapy generally works well. The trouble is patients often drop out from these treatments prematurely. This may be understandable, as the treatment usually requires them to encounter the feared objects or to revisit the traumatic events. Many patients find it difficult and unpleasant.

Vincent solved the problem with an ingenious solution, using a technique called hyperalignment to estimate the patient's voxel patterns for the feared animals using data from other "surrogate" subjects (Haxby et al. 2011, 2020). With enough data, he has demonstrated that it works well. This way, the patients could go through the DecNef-based intervention, without ever having to see any images of animals that they are afraid of (except when we tested them for threat reactions, which was only needed for research rather than clinical purposes).

One important caveat is that in the current studies, subjects did *not* report feeling less afraid when they saw images of the targeted animals. The effect was mainly on their physiological reactions, not their subjective reports of fear. Congruent with a prediction made by Joe Ledoux, perhaps it means that nonconscious treatments can ever only change nonconscious physiological responses (2015). To eliminate the conscious experience of fear, we need to focus directly on mechanisms at that level. Or perhaps, as the methods improve, we will also be able to impact conscious experience using nonconscious DecNef. We will need more experiments to find out.

Regardless, these findings show that nonconscious signals can potentially give us much stronger effects than subliminal priming can. Typically in priming studies, a response is sped up or slowed down by some tens of milliseconds. Here, we robustly changed one's physiological-threat reactions in potentially clinically meaningful ways. Even if the impact on the subjective feelings of fear turns out to be limited, reduction of the physiological-threat reactions can perhaps help patients ease into traditional therapy better. In Taschereau-Dumouchel et al., for the animal categories targeted by DecNef, the physiological-threat reactions, in terms of skin-conductance and amygdala fMRI reactivity, were entirely brought down to baseline level. This was true at least right after the intervention. We do not yet know how long these effects last; we are currently in the process of finding out.

We will further discuss the importance and promise of related clinical applications in Chapter 8.

5.14 Chapter Summary: Partially Global?

The literature on nonconscious priming is vast. It has a long and controversial history. And yet, I've been very selective in covering the relevant studies, to the point that this may look unfair and biased. But the reason is that our question isn't about nonconscious priming per se. The question here is whether consciousness may be associated with higher cognitive functions. The global view says *yes*: consciousness is linked to the prefrontal and parietal cortices, where global coordination and exchange of information take place. Higher cognitive functions should be facilitated by these mechanisms.

The local theorists say *no*: consciousness takes place within the sensory circuitries. Higher cognitive functions are downstream to consciousness. A percept may be nonconscious because it isn't accompanied by the right kind of local dynamics. But the signal may still be able to get out of the local sensory areas to impact the higher cognitive functions downstream.

To answer this question, priming studies are not always the most relevant. In the social cognition literature, many of these studies concern the lack of attention and explicit reflection, rather than the lack of subjective experience per se (Hassin, Uleman, and Bargh 2005). Even when we restrict ourselves to subliminal priming studies, the aim tends to be to show that a function can be influenced by primes that are not consciously perceived. There have also been strong critiques on whether these primes were truly subliminal. Ignoring these critiques is probably not going to help with our progress. Meanwhile, even when we succeed in establishing some subliminal priming effects, they tend to be small. Small effects are easily confused with null effects and are often hard to replicate.

Above all, logically it is not clear how we should interpret these subtle effects. The global theorists can say that although certain functions can operate somewhat nonconsciously, they work much better when we are conscious of the relevant stimuli. Maybe consciousness is always needed for these functions to fully exercise. This may explain why even proponents of the global view like Dehaene seem to have no trouble acknowledging the possibility of a nonconscious working memory and metacognition. Perhaps working-memory representations are more stable, flexible, and effective only when they are conscious.

All the same, it does raise some questions about how these nonconscious higher cognitive effects are even possible. The content of working memory is supposed to be globally accessible. If that's true, how can it be maintained *at all* outside of the workspace? Presumably it means that there must be some other shortcuts for achieving these global functions. But if there are such shortcuts, why do we need the central workspace in the first place? Or perhaps it means that the global workspace isn't so fully global after all. Is it only *part of* a global mechanism, wherein some other parts can operate nonconsciously?

Furthermore, using methods like DecNef, we are beginning to find more powerful forms of nonconscious effects. This may challenge the global view further. Conceptually, nonconscious signals need not be weak by definition. With stronger signals, eventually we may find that higher cognitive functions can be exercised nonconsciously, perhaps even to relatively high degrees of effectiveness.

Despite these threats to the global view, I reviewed some studies showing that consciousness may allow us to more effectively exercise inhibitory and metacognitive functions. The relative advantages provided by consciousness in these cases are not so trivial, especially in the case of metacognition, in the sense that performance capacity was matched. What may be the mechanistic explanation? We will come back to this question in Chapters 7–9.

References

Baars BJ. *A Cognitive Theory of Consciousness*. books.google.com, 1988.

Block N. The Anna Karenina principle and skepticism about unconscious perception. *Philos Phenomenol Res* 2016;**93**:452–459.

Charles L, King J-R, Dehaene S. Decoding the dynamics of action, intention, and error detection for conscious and subliminal stimuli. *J. Neurosci.* 2014;**34**:1158–1170.

Charles L, Van Opstal F, Marti S et al. Distinct brain mechanisms for conscious versus subliminal error detection. *Neuroimage* 2013;**73**:80–94.

Fried I, Katz A, McCarthy G et al. Functional organization of human supplementary motor cortex studied by electrical stimulation. *J Neurosci* 1991;**11**:3656–3666.

van Gaal S, Lamme VAF, Fahrenfort JJ et al. Dissociable brain mechanisms underlying the conscious and unconscious control of behavior. *J Cogn Neurosci* 2011;**23**:91–105.

van Gaal S, Lamme VAF, Ridderinkhof KR. Unconsciously triggered conflict adaptation. *PLOS One* 2010;**5**:e11508.

van Gaal S, Ridderinkhof KR, Fahrenfort JJ et al. Frontal cortex mediates unconsciously triggered inhibitory control. *J Neurosci* 2008;**28**:8053–8062.

van Gaal S, Ridderinkhof KR, Scholte HS et al. Unconscious activation of the prefrontal no-go network. *J Neurosci* 2010;**30**:4143–4150.

Hassin RR, Uleman JS, Bargh JA. *The New Unconscious*. Oxford University Press, 2005.

Haxby JV, Guntupalli JS, Connolly AC et al. A common, high-dimensional model of the representational space in human ventral temporal cortex. *Neuron* 2011;**72**:404–416.

Haxby JV, Guntupalli JS, Nastase SA et al. Hyperalignment: Modeling shared information encoded in idiosyncratic cortical topographies. *Elife* 2020;**9**. https://doi.org/10.7554/eLife.56601.

Hesselmann G, Hebart M, Malach R. Differential BOLD activity associated with subjective and objective reports during "blindsight" in normal observers. *Journal of Neuroscience* 2011;**31**:12936–12944.

Holton NE, Bonner LL, Scott JE et al. The ontogeny of the chin: An analysis of allometric and biomechanical scaling. *Journal of Anatomy* 2015;**226**:549–559.

Huang L, Wang L, Shen W et al. A source for awareness-dependent figure-ground segregation in human prefrontal cortex. *Proc Natl Acad Sci U S A* 2020;**117**:30836–30847.

Jachs B, Blanco MJ, Grantham-Hill S et al. On the independence of visual awareness and metacognition: A signal detection theoretic analysis. *J Exp Psychol Hum Percept Perform* 2015;**41**:269–276.

Jacoby LL, Jones TC, Dolan PO. Two effects of repetition: Support for a dual-process model of know judgments and exclusion errors. *Psychonomic Bulletin & Review* 1998;**5**:705–709.

Kentridge RW, Heywood CA, Weiskrantz L. Attention without awareness in blindsight. *Proceedings of the Royal Society of London Series B: Biological Sciences* 1999;**266**:1805–1811.

Kentridge RW, Heywood CA, Weiskrantz L. Spatial attention speeds discrimination without awareness in blindsight. *Neuropsychologia* 2004;**42**:831–835.

King J-R, Pescetelli N, Dehaene S. Brain mechanisms underlying the brief maintenance of seen and unseen sensory information. *Neuron* 2016;**92**:1122–1134.

Knotts JD, Lau H, Peters MAK. Continuous flash suppression and monocular pattern masking impact subjective awareness similarly. *Atten Percept Psychophys* 2018;**80**:1974–1987.

Koizumi A, Amano K, Cortese A et al. Fear reduction without fear through reinforcement of neural activity that bypasses conscious exposure. *Nat Hum Behav* 2016;**1–6**. https://doi.org/10.1038/s41562-016-0006.

Koizumi A, Maniscalco B, Lau H. Does perceptual confidence facilitate cognitive control? *Atten Percept Psychophys* 2015;**77**:1295–1306.

Kornhuber HH, Deecke L. Changes in the brain potential in voluntary movements and passive movements in man: Readiness potential and reafferent potentials. *Pflugers Arch Gesamte Physiol Menschen Tiere* 1965;**284**:1–17.

Lau HC, Passingham RE. Unconscious activation of the cognitive control system in the human prefrontal cortex. *J Neurosci* 2007;**27**:5805–5811.

Lau HC, Rogers RD, Haggard P et al. Attention to intention. *Science* 2004;**303**:1208–1210.

Lau HC, Rogers RD, Passingham RE. On measuring the perceived onsets of spontaneous actions. *J Neurosci* 2006;**26**:7265–7271.

Lau HC, Rogers RD, Passingham RE. Manipulating the experienced onset of intention after action execution. *J Cogn Neurosci* 2007;**19**:81–90.

LeDoux J. *Anxious: Using the Brain to Understand and Treat Fear and Anxiety.* Penguin, 2015.

Libet B, Gleason CA, Wright EW *et al.* Time of conscious intention to act in relation to onset of cerebral activity (readiness-potential). The unconscious initiation of a freely voluntary act. *Brain* 1983;**106**(Part 3):623–642.

Macmillan NA, Douglas Creelman C. *Detection Theory: A User's Guide.* Psychology Press, 2004.

Maniscalco B, Castaneda OG, Odegaard B et al. The metaperceptual function: Exploring dissociations between confidence and task performance with type 2 psychometric curves. *PsyArxiv* 2020. https://doi.org/10.31234/osf.io/5qrjn.

Naccache L, Dehaene S. Unconscious semantic priming extends to novel unseen stimuli. *Cognition* 2001;**80**:215–229.

Nikolov S, Rahnev DA, Lau HC. Probabilistic model of onset detection explains paradoxes in human time perception. *Front Psychol* 2010;**1**:37.

Persaud N, Cowey A. Blindsight is unlike normal conscious vision: Evidence from an exclusion task. *Conscious Cogn* 2008;17:1050–1055.

Persaud N, Davidson M, Maniscalco B et al. Awareness-related activity in prefrontal and parietal cortices in blindsight reflects more than superior visual performance. *Neuroimage* 2011;58:605–611.

Persaud N, Lau H. Direct assessment of qualia in a blindsight participant. *Consciousness and Cognition* 2008;17:1046–1049.

Peters MAK, Lau H. Human observers have optimal introspective access to perceptual processes even for visually masked stimuli. *Elife* 2015;4:e09651.

Rahnev DA, Huang E, Lau H. Subliminal stimuli in the near absence of attention influence top-down cognitive control. *Atten Percept Psychophys* 2012;74:521–532.

Robinson Z, Maley CJ, Piccinini G. Is consciousness a spandrel? *Journal of the American Philosophical Association* 2015;1:365–383.

Romo R, Schultz W. Neuronal activity preceding self-initiated or externally timed arm movements in area 6 of monkey cortex. *Exp Brain Res* 1987;67:656–662.

Schurger A, Sitt JD, Dehaene S. An accumulator model for spontaneous neural activity prior to self-initiated movement. *Proc Natl Acad Sci U S A* 2012;109:e2904–e2913.

Scott RB, Samaha J, Chrisley R et al. Prevailing theories of consciousness are challenged by novel cross-modal associations acquired between subliminal stimuli. *Cognition* 2018;175:169–185.

Shea N, Frith CD. The global workspace needs metacognition. *Trends Cogn Sci* 2019;23:560–571.

Shibata K, Watanabe T, Sasaki Y et al. Perceptual learning incepted by decoded fMRI neurofeedback without stimulus presentation. *Science* 2011;334:1413–1415.

Soon CS, Brass M, Heinze H-J et al. Unconscious determinants of free decisions in the human brain. *Nat Neurosci* 2008;11:543–545.

Taschereau-Dumouchel V, Cortese A, Chiba T et al. Towards an unconscious neural reinforcement intervention for common fears. *Proceedings of the National Academy of Sciences* 2018;115:3470–3475.

Trübutschek D, Marti S, Dehaene S. Temporal-order information can be maintained in non-conscious working memory. *Sci Rep* 2019;9:6484.

Trübutschek D, Marti S, Ojeda A et al. A theory of working memory without consciousness or sustained activity. *Elife* 2017;6. https://doi.org/10.7554/eLife.23871.

Trübutschek D, Marti S, Ueberschär H et al. Probing the limits of activity-silent non-conscious working memory. *Proc Natl Acad Sci U S A* 2019;116:14358–14367.

Tsushima Y, Sasaki Y, Watanabe T. Greater disruption due to failure of inhibitory control on an ambiguous distractor. *Science* 2006;314:1786–1788.

Watanabe T, Sasaki Y, Shibata K et al. Advances in fMRI real-time neurofeedback. *Trends Cogn Sci* 2017;21:12;997–1010.

Wegner DM. Précis of the illusion of conscious will. *Behav Brain Sci* 2004;**27**:649–659; discussion 659–692.

Zhang X, Zhaoping L, Zhou T et al. Neural activities in V1 create a bottom-up saliency map. *Neuron* 2012;**73**:183–192.

6

A Centrist Manifesto

6.1 Striking a Balance

The main goal of this chapter is to take stock of what we have reviewed so far, and to assess the broader theoretical implications. We have covered the first three of the five main issues introduced in Chapter 1: the neural correlates of consciousness (NCC), the relationship between attention and consciousness, and the functions of consciousness. The remaining two issues concern whether animals and robots can be conscious. To address them we need to make some theoretical generalizations. Fortunately, the previous chapters provide some constraints for what an adequate theory should look like.

Overall, neither the global nor local view works well. Instead the evidence points to a synthesis. The key findings from the previous chapters will be summarized here.

Throughout, I will also introduce some new empirical and theoretical considerations, especially in Sections 6.6–6.9.

6.2 Troubles for Global Theories

The global view faces several empirical challenges. The first is that when experimental confounders are controlled for, the activations in the prefrontal and parietal cortices are not as widespread as we once thought (Chapter 2). In some cases null findings were overinterpreted: when reports were not required, there were actually still clearly observable activity in the prefrontal and parietal cortices; this depends on the measurement methods. But it is fair to say that the activity becomes more subtle under these conditions. Likewise, controlling for task-performance capacity reduces activity in these regions. These findings suggest that global broadcast may largely support task performance and reports, rather than subjective experience per se.

Congruent with this interpretation is the fact that information represented in the workspace does not always come with subjective experience. As discussed in Chapter 5, Dehaene and colleagues have themselves been studying

In Consciousness We Trust. Hakwan Lau, Oxford University Press. © Hakwan Lau 2022.
DOI: 10.1093/oso/9780198856771.003.0007

nonconscious working memory by applying visual masks to the relevant stimuli. But even for typical, unmasked stimuli, there aren't always strong perceptual experiences during the working-memory delay. For example, if one has to memorize a visual pattern for 10 seconds, one may invoke visual imagery of the pattern during the delay. But this visual imagery is not generally confused with the subjective experience of conscious perception. More importantly, some people never experience vivid visual imagery—a condition known as aphantasia (Zeman, Dewar, and Della Sala 2015). And yet they seem to have no trouble doing these working-memory tasks. According to global theories, during the working-memory delay, the information is maintained in part by workspace mechanisms. Why does the content of working memory not "leak out" into consciousness, so that we subjectively perceive it as if the stimulus is right in front of us?

And then other nonconscious stimuli also seem to reach the prefrontal cortex and influence higher cognitive functions, as shown in subliminal priming studies (Chapter 5). Just why don't these stimuli lead to conscious experience, given that they have reached the workspace?

Similarly, the global view may have troubles accounting for certain perceptual phenomena such as blindsight. If the explanation is that such information fails to reach the workspace, one needs to account for how they can lead to task performance at sometimes above 80% correct (in, e.g., two-choice discriminations). What may be the mechanisms that allow a signal to influence behavior so strongly, and yet bypass the workspace?

Dehaene and colleagues may answer that there could be a nonconscious channel operating *in parallel*, which accounts for blindsight and other nonconscious behavior. But when this parallel model was formally compared against *hierarchical* models, the latter performed better (Chapter 3 Section 3.8). This is congruent with the fact that conscious and nonconscious processing both depend on the very same early sensory areas (Chapter 2). There are no exclusive early sensory pathways for conscious perception only. Instead, the difference between conscious and nonconscious processing seems to depend on some specific late-stage process (the hierarchical model). It is unlikely that such a late-stage process is the global workspace itself. That's because the workspace is meant to be functionally important. If the difference in late-stage process is associated with such a big functional difference, we would expect consciousness to come with very many functional advantages. And yet it doesn't. To the extent there are such advantages, the most likely candidates seem to be metacognition, and to a lesser extent, inhibitory control (Chapter 5). But global broadcast functions are sometimes thought to be independent from metacognition (Dehaene, Lau, and Kouider 2017).

Not only are there cases where functionally strong perceptual signals aren't conscious, the opposite scenario also seems possible. One example is peripheral vision, or subjective perception in the unattended background (Chapter 4). There, the information seems not to be processed well in the central workspace. People are poor at reporting the details, or they miss salient events altogether. And yet, subjectively, there seems to be an inflated sense of experience; the unattended background looks more vivid than expected, given how poorly the details are actually represented.

Finally, lesion studies also put some pressure on the global view. Prefrontal and parietal lesions do not seem to abolish broadcast. There are important caveats to keep in mind as we interpret lesion data; they do not straightforwardly tell us whether certain brain areas are "necessary" (see Sections 2.3 and 3.2). However, despite this caveat, it is true that prefrontal lesions impair metacognition and response inhibition. But these patients continue to be able to perform many other perceptual and cognitive tasks at a high level, as if the global broadcast mechanism remains unaffected.

These are not the only problems for the global view. As we'll see in the next chapters, the view also predicts that very simple computer programs and robots may be conscious. That may be considered implausible by some. But for now, the evidence based on human data may suffice.

6.3 Rejoinders?

The global theorist can perhaps bluntly deny the relevance of lesion studies. Perhaps the lack of impact on workspace functions is because of the resilience of the frontoparietal network. When one part is damaged another can take over (as discussed in Chapter 3). It is also true that inhibitory control can be considered a higher cognitive function related to workspace mechanisms.

They can also point to the paucity of decisive evidence against the parallel channels model. Maniscalco and Lau (2016) was just a single study, and its conclusion awaits to be confirmed by more studies directly comparing models, with different datasets. Likewise, they can write-off subliminal priming studies because most of those effects are small. Perhaps the global workspace is needed to exercise those cognitive functions fully.

But I'm not sure how a global theorist can satisfactorily address the apparent double dissociation constituted by the cases of working memory and peripheral vision. By double dissociation, I'm referring to the fact that information represented in the workspace is sometimes nonconscious (e.g., visual working memory, especially in aphantasics), and that conscious experiences sometimes outstrip information represented in the workspace (as in cases of peripheral or unattended perception).

Regarding peripheral vision or perception in the unattended background, perhaps the global theorist can say that subjective experience isn't really inflated. They can insist that the experience is actually just as sparse as the represented content, only that we are mistaken about the experience. In Chapter 4 we discussed that the subjective appearance of richness may not be universal. But at least some subjects feel that they see more than they have access to, at least under some conditions. For the globalist reply to work, we need to deny that they are right about their own experiences. We need to say that subjects are only aware of what their global workspace can represent, but not more, regardless of what they think. This leads to a conceptual question: to what extent can we really be mistaken about our conscious experiences? If we honestly feel that the peripheral perception is rich, how wrong can we be? Or consider this alternative: if we honestly feel a blinding headache, what does it matter if someone says we are mistaken?

These problems should be considered in the context of the frontal and parietal activations found in studies of consciousness. The current domination of the global view has much to do with the supposedly widespread and robust nature of these activations. But in the light of the new findings of much more subtle activity, when confounders were controlled for, it may be time to revisit whether our initial enthusiasm for the global view is justified. To the extent that some fronto-parietal mechanisms are critical for consciousness, it may be much more specific than a widespread broadcast mechanism. If we detach the notion of consciousness from such a general functional network, the problem of the double dissociation discussed may be easier to address. Perhaps global broadcast does happen often for consciously perceived stimuli, but only as a typical downstream consequence rather than as a constitutive mechanism.

6.4 Troubles for Local Theories

The local view likewise cannot account for the present evidence. While local theorists argue that the activity in the prefrontal and parietal cortices was reduced when report and attention were controlled for, the activity was not completely gone. In particular, this seems to depend heavily on the measurement method. Using invasive methods at high resolution, the measured activity remained strong even under these controls (Chapter 2). This suggests that the activity involved in conscious perception goes beyond the local sensory circuits.

Furthermore, it is unclear if the local activity itself survives the control of similar confounders. When task-performance capacity was controlled for, null results were also obtained in the visual cortex (Section 2.11). As in the case of the prefrontal cortex, we should not overinterpret individual null results. But it does raise the question of whether activity in the visual cortex really just drives basic visual processing for potential task performance, or subjective experience per se. This worry is highlighted by the phenomenon of nonconscious binocular rivalry. Invisible stimuli leading to such rivalry seem to activate the visual cortex just as visible stimuli do (Section 2.10). So, early sensory activity alone is not always associated with subjective experience.

Similarly, regarding the case of unattended or peripheral perception, the localist argument against the global view may not work well or may even backfire. Local theorists appeal to the fact that subjective experience seems rich, at least to some subjects. Because prefrontal mechanisms are supposed to have limited processing capacity, they are thought to be "overflown" by the richness of experience. But there are two problems with this argument. The first is that the role of the prefrontal cortex may not be to "duplicate" the sensory information. Rather, it may just monitor and redirect information in the sensory cortices, using something akin to indexing mechanisms. If so, the putative limited capacity may not be an issue.

The second problem is more directly challenging for the local view itself: it is unclear if the early sensory cortices represent perceptual information detailed enough to account for the subjective richness. In particular, although the level of reported richness may vary across people, it seems relatively stable within a person. However, early sensory activity is modulated strongly by attention. Even holding the spatial focus constant, a mere change in the task is enough to robustly change early sensory activity. And yet the subjective experience of richness does not seem to change nearly as much (Chapter 4).

Overall, there seems to be many instances in which the content reflected by early visual activity just does not seem to match with the content of conscious perception (Section 2.5). This is especially a problem if we focus on a specific local view, according to which the NCC involves a specific visual area (e.g., (feedback to) V1). The different sensory areas all exist for important functional reasons. Depending on the stimuli and context, is it likely that perception will capitalize on all possible sensory resources under different situations. At times, the perceptual phenomenology is probably too complex to be described by just content at one level (Section 4.12).

As with the global view, some local theories also tend to implicitly adopt the parallel channels model. In order to account for strong nonconscious perceptual processes (e.g., in blindsight), some alternative pathways presumably need to be invoked. But as we mentioned earlier in Section 6.2, the parallel channels model is not well-supported empirically, compared to the hierarchical model.

One way to avoid this problem may be to think of feedforward processes (e.g., from V1 to MT) as nonconscious, such that feedback (e.g., from MT back to V1) may constitute the later stage process within a hierarchy. This would give us a hierarchical interpretation of Lamme's recurrency theory. However, the evidence in support of the role of feedback processes in conscious perception is confounded by task-performance capacity and attention. That is, when feedback processes were supposedly disrupted, not only was subjective experience abolished, processing capacity was also much weakened (Manita et al. 2015; Peters et al. 2017a). As such, it is unclear if feedforward processes alone can lead to nonconscious perceptual signals which are as strong as those supported by recurrency. This makes the hierarchical interpretation problematic because the late stage in the model is not supposed to contribute directly to task performance itself.

Let's assume, for the sake of argument, that there can be strong nonconscious perceptual processes without feedback. One problem is that this version of a local view makes rather implausible predictions about the functions of consciousness. As suggested by van Gaal and Lamme, the nonconscious feedforward signal can propagate into the prefrontal cortex to exercise higher cognitive functions (Section 5.5). This may seem compatible with studies of subliminal priming. However, according to this local view, these signals can be very strong. But subliminal priming effects are invariably weak. The local theorist will have to predict that at least under some conditions, there can be nonconscious effects on these higher cognitive functions that are just as strong and robust as conscious cases. Given current findings, this seems improbable. I am aware of no reports so far on *fully preserved* higher cognitive functions when conscious perception of the relevant stimuli is abolished (via blocking of feedback processing). Overall, it seems much more plausible that feedback processing in the sensory cortices is important for perception in general, but not specifically for subjective experience per se.

Finally, local theorists often criticize the global view based on lesion cases, but their own view is in fact just as problematic in this context, if not more. It is true that in blindsight, the abolishment of visual awareness happens after lesions to the primary cortex. However, blindsight is most clearly established for static stimuli. By magnetically stimulating the remaining extrastriate areas, researchers successfully induced subjective experience of motion in a blindsight patient, where the corresponding V1 was absent (Section 2.4). There have also been reports about patients experiencing hallucinations after damage to early visual areas (Lau and Brown 2019). Vivid visual mental imagery is also possible after V1 damage (Bridge et al. 2012). In subjects from the general population, V1 itself also seems relatively deactivated in dreams (Braun et al. 1998).

6.5 Contrivance

The localists can insist that strong subliminal modulation of higher cognitive functions is in fact possible. Maybe the problem is just that we have not *yet* figured out how to truly selectively abolish feedback to early sensory areas, without compromising the overall perceptual signal, in order to induce such strong nonconscious percepts. In the absence of positive evidence, I'm not so sure how plausible a hierarchical interpretation of their theory is. But perhaps, like the global theorists, they can also deny the current evidence against the parallel channel model, on the grounds that more studies are needed.

Still, the burden of proof should be on the local theorists to demonstrate that their early sensory correlates are not merely driven by the confounder of performance capacity. As it currently stands, the confounder seems to be the most likely explanation. That is, early sensory activity drives perception, but not subjective experience per se.

As to prefrontal activity surviving various confounds, the local theorists can insist that such activity is weak. They can also argue that evidence for their causal involvement in consciousness (e.g., from lesion and stimulation) is not so strong. But the analysis of the NCC is a logical matter. It shouldn't be based on the *impression* of what looks more obvious given our current methods. We should not treat weak effects as nonexistent, especially if we have independent reasons to expect such effects to be weak, given the anatomy and physiology of the prefrontal cortex (Section 3.11).

However, I concede that prefrontal involvement in subjective perceptual experience is in fact subtle. So the localists may be right that the global position is not sound. Subjective experience may not always constitutively depend on something as involved as global broadcast. But it does not mean that the localists are right in writing off the prefrontal cortex entirely either.

Another difficult challenge for local theorists is the issue of content mismatch (Section 2.5). Again, like the global theorists, the localists can perhaps insist that whatever content is reflected by early sensory activity, that is in fact the content of conscious perception. Any discrepancy may be due to the subjects' mistaking what they truly perceive. But some of these illusions are so vivid and easy for all of us to see (Section 2.5). To say we can be so consistently wrong about our own experiences just seems rather unconvincing.

Above all, it should be clear that the localist NCC candidate of feedback to V1 isn't very promising (Hupé et al. 2001; Huang et al. 2020). There are clear cases of occurrence of subjective experience in the absence of V1 activity. To say that we are mistaken about some details of our perceptual content is one thing; it's a different matter to say that subjects regularly misconstrues themselves as having perceptual experiences when there are actually none (according to one's assumed notion of NCC). Therefore, to the extent a local view is plausible *at all*, the likely NCC candidate is probably extrastriate local activity, rather than feedback to V1.

6.6 Two Opposing Dogmas

The above leaves us with a conundrum. Philosophers like Ned Block sometimes favor the local recurrency view, I think largely because "recurrency" gives a flavor that it is a special kind of biological activity. They are hoping to look for that unique physical substrate, to be identified with the inexplicable characters of subjective experience (or to otherwise explain them away somehow).

Given that V1 is unlikely to be truly part of the NCC, in order to retain the notion of "recurrency," perhaps one can hold that visual awareness constitutively depends on interactions between the prefrontal cortex and extrastriate areas (Huang et al. 2020). This view may not be so implausible. However, this will not strictly be a *local* view.

More importantly, the problem is that there is actually nothing magical about recurrent activity. Cortical areas are bidirectionally connected. Recurrency is likely just the normal way different areas work together effectively. Many artificial neural networks also employ feedback architectures.

So, if the local NCC is just extrastriate activity rather than interregional recurrency, what is so special about such activity? For truly local theorists, the downstream impact (e.g., to the prefrontal cortex) of such activity shouldn't matter. What is so special about these signals within an area, which may not even end up having any downstream impact at all?

One extreme answer is that there is nothing special. Any physical objects that can signal or represent information are conscious to some extent (Chalmers 1996; Roelofs 2019). Because even a single photon can arguably "represent" some minimal amount of information, the view implies that pretty much all physical things can be conscious. This rather far-fetched view, called *panpsychism*, remains mostly a matter of philosophical conjecture. As such, I hesitate to even mention it here. However, although the view lacks serious scientific attention, it has generated considerable public excitement in recent years. In Chapter 8 I will discuss some disadvantages of this position. It would most likely disallow us from making useful connections with much of the rest of academia. And then in Chapter 9 we will finally revisit this "problem" again.

A more scientifically acceptable position may be biopsychism (Godfrey-Smith 2016). On a strong version, all and only all biological organisms are conscious. On a weaker version, only biological organisms are conscious; some aren't. Let us focus on this latter, weaker version of biopsychism. According to this view, perhaps the need to self-regulate metabolic activity is an important ingredient for consciousness, but downstream impact on information processing is not. That is, if we replace those extrastriate spiking activities with silicon chips and electrodes exactly mimicking the outgoing signals, the subjective experience may well be gone (or at least drastically different). The correct substrate has to be "biological."

I suspect that some cognitive neuroscientists will find this biopsychic view puzzling, if not downright absurd. The modern approach to studying the brain is to think of it as an organ for information processing. We analogize brains with computers. Brain mechanisms exist because they *function* in a certain way. But all the same, some of the most prominent local theorists do endorse biopsychism. Arguably, this is the logical end point of local theories: effective information processing ultimately depends on the global context of the entire system. If local theorists want to have nothing to do with that, their view is unavoidably at odds with the very premise of cognitive neuroscience. They are essentially skeptics of the information processing approach to understanding the mind.

One motivation for biopsychism may be that the obvious alternatives may not seem so appealing. Some local theorists may argue against *functionalism*, the idea that subjective experience is determined by the roles played by the relevant substrates in informational processing. Specifically, one view that has been systematically criticized is what we can call *long-arm* functionalism (Block 1990). According to the view, consciousness is determined by what is targeted or represented by the system *in the environment*. For example, some brain activity is about an apple in front of us because it tracks and is about the apple. To the extent that the activity tracks the apple, and that it signals the rest of the system to refer to *that* apple, the activity plays the relevant "long-arm" functional roles. Long-arm functionalism isn't so attractive because it might be thought to equate consciousness with behavioral functions. It is all about how the brain or a physical system can relate to objects out there, and act accordingly. Arguably, nonconscious perceptual processes can also play these long-arm functional roles. Also, the same represented apple may cause different subjective experiences, depending on contexts, perspectives, etc.

To take it to the "globalist" extreme, some versions of functionalism may further postulate that language is needed to relate to these objects in the environment in a truly meaningful way. To be conscious of the objects, we may need to be able to form explicit thoughts about them, and to potentially articulate such thoughts to others and ourselves. This kind of view is often criticized for overintellectualizing consciousness. That is, it misconstrues the sheer occurrence of simple subjective experience as something that requires sophisticated forms of cognition and intelligence.

Fortunately, not all versions of functionalism are of the long-arm type, nor do they require overintellectualization. In fact, most modern cognitive neuroscientists don't endorse such views. All they hold is that information processing is all that matters; the hardware, that is the physical substrate, doesn't really matter, *to the extent that the relevant algorithms are correctly implemented*. As such, the "long-arm" functional roles are only a small part of the story. How these neural representations function *internally*, that is, how they impact downstream cognition, also matters. We can call this view internal functionalism. But sometimes I will just call it functionalism, because long-arm functionalism is a just strawman in this specific context.

This broader notion of (internal) functionalism can sit comfortably between the two extreme dogmas: that consciousness is either something to be equated with sophisticated cognition, or something physically characterized such that it may not do much cognitively at all. Neither is right. But the functional role played by conscious neural representations may not be to broadcast globally to the entire system, in order to lead to *more* cognition in general. It is likely something more specific and modest. So this would avoid much of the problems faced by the global view. But still, whatever functions it involves, it would likely have some specific impact on downstream cognition and behavior. That would explain the subtle involvement of the prefrontal cortex in studies of conscious perception.

Nor do I write-off the concerns of biopsychists entirely; perhaps something about the physical substrates does matter too. I will try to account for this latter intuition in Chapter 9, within a functionalist framework.

6.7 Varieties of Centrism

What may be a functionalist account of consciousness that does not equate consciousness with global broadcast? There are many variants that would more or less qualify (Brown, Lau, and LeDoux 2019). For example, I am sympathetic to Axel Cleeremans' self-organizing metarepresentational account (Cleeremans et al. 2020). According to the view, subjective experience arises when the brain learns to represent its own sensory states for the purpose of hierarchical control of perceptual information and action. That is, the information in the early sensory states are being redescribed at a later stage, for self-monitoring purposes.

This view shares some similarity with a broad class of philosophical theories known as higher-order views. One influential version is David Rosenthal's higher-order thought theory (2005), which we will discuss briefly in Chapter 7. One key characteristic of this family of views is that the relevant higher-order mechanism is meant to be much more specific than global broadcast. To the extent that it is functionally important, it may only serve a rather narrow range of purposes. It may not strengthen the relevant internal perceptual signal or make it more stable, sustained, or complex. In fact, Rosenthal himself argued that consciousness may come with little or no added utility. To some, this may sound extreme and implausible. I myself also do not share this "minimalist" view on the functions of consciousness. But in contrast with global views, we can see why this is a relatively moderate, "centrist" position. Like a globalist position this is a functionalist account, and yet like a local view it does not assume that consciousness is just the same as more powerful and effective cognition in general. This would fit much better than the evidence reviewed in Chapter 5.

Of note is the fact that Richard Brown is also a higher-order theorist (LeDoux and Brown 2017), and yet he is more sympathetic to biopsychism than to functionalism (Brown 2012). According to such a view, perhaps the relevant self-monitoring (i.e., higher-order) mechanisms need to be implemented biologically. This highlights the fact that within this space between the two theoretical extremes, there are really many options available. To be a "centrist" is to resist the global and local extremes. But this does not on its own commit the theorist to functionalism or biopsychism; although most "centrists," including myself, are functionalists (in the broad, internal sense described in the Section 6.6). Like I said in the previous section, we will address some biopsychic intuitions again in Chapter 9.

Instead of doing a detailed comparison between all possible "centrist" positions, I will instead highlight two sets of considerations, one empirical and one theoretical, inspired by current models of artificial intelligence. Together, they put further constraints on what a plausible centrist theory should look like.

6.8 Metacognition & Detection

In Chapters 3 and 4, we pointed out that metacognition seems relevant to subjective experience. In a sense, we could consider this a brute fact: we identified areas of the prefrontal cortex as important for consciousness, mostly based on findings from neuroimaging (Chapter 2). When these areas were targeted by magnetic stimulation and chemical inactivation, or if they were lesioned, we found that metacognition was also affected (Chapter 3). In particular, at least in some studies, this was specific to perceptual rather than mnemonic metacognition.

However, that two functions employ a common brain region may not mean much; we only have so many brain regions at this coarse-grained level. But conceptually there may be a deeper link between metacognition and consciousness too. If one consciously perceives something, it seems to make little sense to say that one has zero confidence about any aspect of the percept. Of course, sometimes we *see* something without being able to recognize what the object is. But at least we should be fairly sure that something is *seen*, not *heard*. If one is truly unsure what modality the percept involves, perhaps it is doubtful whether there is any subjective experience at all.

That is to say, having a subjective experience seems to involve *detecting* the presence of some signal in the relevant sensory modality (Fleming 2020). This is not to suggest they are one and the same. But incidentally, as we mentioned in Section 3.9, lesions to the prefrontal cortex can impair behavior in some detection tasks too. In peripheral or unattended vision, we also know that subjects use a relatively liberal detection criterion—a phenomenon I called "inflation." In Chapter 4, I speculated that the underlying mechanism may be in the prefrontal cortex, which we know is important for perceptual metacognition.

Why are metacognition and detection linked? Theoretically, they do not have to be. If the task is discrimination between two stimulus alternatives (whether an apple or an orange is presented), one can just compare the two relevant signals against each other. Whether they are both strong or weak does not strictly matter; we only need to know the direction and magnitude of the *difference* between the two signals. If the difference is large, we rate high confidence; if the difference is small, we rate low confidence. But empirically we know that human subjects often do not do that. Unless they are overtrained on a specific task, when asked to rate confidence, they often resort to using the detectability of the stimulus as a heuristic (Maniscalco, Peters, and Lau 2016).

For example, Megan Peters and Aurelio Cortese have conducted neuroimaging studies to test this. I was involved in both of their studies, but they were conducted independently using different methods. In both cases, we found that the internal brain signals contributing to confidence ratings were basically just the amount of total detectable signals for the stimuli, rather than the difference between the relevant signals (Cortese et al. 2016; Peters et al. 2017c).

Why do human subjects use such a strategy, which seems highly suboptimal? Essentially, they are neglecting useful information. The exact mechanism remains an open topic for current research (Miyoshi and Lau 2020). But in any case, it points to a strong empirical link between detection and metacognition. Somehow, when asked to give confidence ratings, people resort to heuristics based largely on detectability of the stimuli. Arguably, both metacognition and detection are also conceptually related to subjective experiences. In Chapter 5 we also highlighted metacognition as one of the possible key functions of consciousness, maybe the most plausible one so far, given the limited evidence we have. It would be a nice feature of a theory of consciousness to be able to say something about how they are all tied together.

6.9 Predictive Coding & Generative Adversarial Networks

In recent years, *predictive coding* has become a trendy phrase. This has led some authors to speculate that it may have something to do with consciousness. But sometimes the phrase just refers to the fact that the brain can generate or modulate internal sensory representations in ways not entirely driven by external input (Cao 2020). In this sense, the notion is nothing new. With a few exceptions (Gibson 1968), most modern psychologists agree that perception involves top-down mechanisms of some sort.

More specifically, one idea is that external sensory inputs may be assessed with respect to the endogenously generated expectation. If our expectations are not violated, we learn nothing new; not much is worth signaling. In contrast, "prediction errors" are very much worth signaling downstream, as they carry novel information. But even this more specific notion of predictive coding is actually rather general; some have long considered it a "standard" view on how the brain works. This is not to say there is no controversy around how it works (Aitchison and Lengyel 2017). But there has also been numerous reports showing that stimuli not consciously perceived can drive this type of predictive process as well, at least to some extent (Iijima and Sakai 2014; Chang et al. 2016; Parras et al. 2017; Meijs et al. 2018; Nourski et al. 2018; Rowe, Tsuchiya, and Garrido 2020). So, it is not clear if "predictive coding" has anything specific to do with consciousness per se.

One interesting fact about predictive coding is that it is not entirely trivial to implement using artificial neural networks. Until recently, most pattern recognition networks adopted a feedforward-only architecture. This is not because computer scientists do not recognize the benefits of predictive coding, of which there are many. The problem is that building a network model to accurately produce top-down generations requires a lot of training time and data.

One solution has been extremely influential within the artificial intelligence community. In generative adversarial networks (GANs), a "generator" could take high level conceptual inputs (e.g., the notion of a "cat") and come up with a corresponding pictorial representation (Goodfellow, Bengio, and Courville 2016). A "discriminator" learns to distinguish between these pictorial outputs from the "generator," and actual images in the world. Both components are easy to build using current technology. In particular, the "discriminator" is akin to a simple pattern classification network. Just like the way a simple facial recognition algorithm can categorize faces as male or female, the "discriminator" makes simple binary decisions on some image inputs to classify input as "real" or "self-generated" (Figure 6.1).

What is interesting is that when we pit the two networks against each other, both networks quickly learn to do their jobs well. That is, we can think of the generator's job is to create "forgeries" (i.e., internally generated pictures that are close enough to the real ones). If it succeeds in fooling the discriminator, it counts as a win. Likewise, the discriminator's "goal" is to catch such forgeries. With these simple and competitive goals set up, both networks can be trained efficiently.

This GANs architecture may be related to consciousness in several ways. First, it has been suggested on theoretical grounds that a discriminator-like mechanism may reside within the prefrontal cortex (Gershman 2019; Lau 2019). In support of this claim, there has been physiological evidence (Mendoza-Halliday and Martinez-Trujillo 2017) showing that neurons in the dorsolateral prefrontal cortex can distinguish between external perceptual content and endogenous generation of the same content (i.e., maintenance of the same information during working-memory delay). This is interesting because holding an image in working memory tends to induce somewhat similar activity in the early visual areas as normal perception (Harrison and

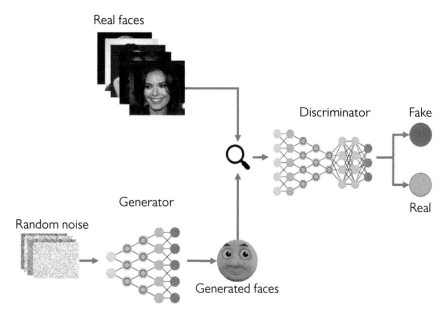

Figure 6.1 GANs architecture

Tong 2009). So, the difference in conscious experience between the two conditions, working memory and perception, may be captured by a discriminator-like mechanism in the prefrontal cortex.

Relatedly, a postdoc in my lab, Taylor Webb, has recently trained a GANs model to perform a simple perceptual task. He found that the discriminator can be "repurposed" to perform metacognitive functions (i.e., generation of confidence ratings) with minimal impact to the discriminator's performance. On the assumption that metacognition and consciousness are linked, perhaps a discriminator-like mechanism can contribute to both too. Although this work is yet to be published, the finding may not be surprising to those familiar to GANs. The discriminator naturally contains rich statistical information about the relevant stimuli, for otherwise it would not be able to do its job.

In Chapter 7, we will put forward a theory describing how human consciousness may critically depend on a discriminator-like mechanism within a GANs-like architecture.

6.10 Interlude: Some Loose Ends

Because this chapter in part summarizes findings discussed in previous chapters, I will not provide a detailed recap here. In brief, we have argued against both the global and local views. We have outlined what developing a plausible synthesis involves. We need to resist the localist temptation, to fall into extreme positions such as panpsychism. To provide a meaningful mechanistic explanation, we need some form of functionalist account. But we must also avoid equating consciousness with basic cognitive functions such as global control or broadcast. As far as subjective experiences are concerned, such a view is not really compatible with available data.

Instead, we want a view that can account for the relatively subtle activity in the prefrontal cortex during conscious perception, as well as the functional advantages provided—which is far more specific than a globalist may expect. This should in turn elucidate how inflation works, as well as to explain the links between conscious perception, metacognition, and detection. Ideally, this should also take into consideration how the relevant prefrontal mechanisms may relate to current models of predictive coding. Specifically, we should try to take into account the electrophysiological evidence that the prefrontal cortex seems to play a role in discriminating between self-generated and externally triggered perceptual signals.

This agenda is based on my review of the empirical literature so far. Like in any review, I cannot claim that I'm entirely unbiased. All I can say is that my various arguments are based on different evidence and considerations. To the extent that these separate arguments point to a converging conclusion, it is, I hope, not so easy to argue against all of them at once. However, there is indeed one crucial sticking point. My experience in debating with critics is that once this point is accepted, all the counter-arguments will fall like dominoes. But it also means that if this point is challenged, a lot would be at stake.

What is this crucial sticking point? My overall take on the empirical literature depends critically on the notion of task-performance capacity confounders. Performance *capacity* is not performance itself. Even when there is no task, such as in some binocular rivalry experiments, there is this same hidden problem of difference in sheer internal processing signal strength (Chapter 2). Some may say: but this *is* consciousness. My reply is mostly based on the counterexample of blindsight: sometimes performance comes with no corresponding subjective experience.

Understanding this potential dissociation between task-performance capacity and subjective experience may be the cornerstone for the entire thesis here. But some have challenged whether blindsight truly exists (Phillips 2020). There may be subjective experience unreported by the patients, because the experience is so impoverished and unusual. I agree that some "diagnosed" patients may not have "true" blindsight. Even for those who do, it may not be present under all conditions. But for some well-studied patients, for certain stimuli (e.g., static, low-contrast gratings) very meticulous controls have been performed (Cowey 2010). Given the nature of patient studies, this is in fact one of the better-established phenomena within neuropsychology. Accordingly, Matthias Michel and I have responded to Ian Phillips's recent arguments against the existence of blindsight in detail (Michel and Lau 2021).

The important key point is that blindsight does not need to occur very often. If it happens convincingly on rare occasions, the phenomenon establishes the conceptual and empirical *possibility* of the dissociation between task-performance capacity and subjective experience.

Perhaps Phillips' arguments should be considered within a broader context too, in which he has argued against the possibility of nonconscious perception in general (Peters et al. 2017b). This debate largely hinges on how *perception* is defined. Specifically, our concern here is not whether there can be nonconscious perception that takes place *at the personal level*. If one does not consciously see something, there's perhaps an argument to be made that one does not, as an agent, "perceive" the relevant object, in some meaningful sense. But to deny any kind of nonconscious perceptual *process* would entail that all perceptually relevant processes in the brain are by definition conscious, which seems highly implausible.

Accordingly, my argument for task-performance capacity confounders rests on just this fact: that some meaningful information processing can take place nonconsciously. This kind of dissociation between subjective experience and information processing is also found in other classic cases in neuropsychology (e.g., amnesia and split-brain patients; LeDoux, Michel, and Lau 2020). So, consciousness just isn't as simple as effective information processing of any kind. With this, we establish the need to control for this confounder. This realization renders most current popular claims about the NCC problematic and forces us to accept a centrist position.

But there is another problem: how do we control for the confounder? I suggest that we can match performance levels in some tasks. But then the question arises as to what tasks are most relevant. For example, in Lau and Passingham (2006), the stimuli were a square and a rhombus (i.e., a square tilted by 45 degrees). The subjects discriminated between the two. It may seem fair that we match performance levels in this discrimination task. But why not a detection task (of identifying stimulus present or absence)? When task performance in discrimination is matched, are we sure detection performance is also matched? If not, do we not leave open a detection-task-performance confounder?

This is a deep and complicated issue. The processing sensitivity for a stimulus can be assessed in different "dimensions" (e.g., detectability, and

discriminability based on various features). Ideally, we match basic performance in all these different tasks. To the extent that the relationship between
sensitivities in these dimensions don't change, matching it on one task is sufficient. But the relationship may not be empirically constant, which can lead
to some serious complications. That said, matching performance in one obviously relevant task dimension is in any case far better than no match whatsoever. So, this is perhaps the bottom line: just because a confounder is difficult
to deal with doesn't mean that we should give up dealing with it altogether. We
do it as best as we can.

A different issue also concerns the NCC. My view may come across as giving
the prefrontal cortex too much attention. In the beginning of Chapter 3, I justified this focus. Unlike local theorists, our intention is not to write-off other
areas as irrelevant. Many other areas, including subcortical regions, may also
be highly important. My point here is only that the prefrontal cortex may be
one of the many important pieces of the puzzle.

That said, from here, the theory I will introduce will be grounded in what we
have reviewed so far. As such, it may neglect the possible roles played by some
other brain regions and circuits, including, for example, the claustrum and the
thalamus (including, especially, the pulvinar). Perhaps to build a theory that
usefully captures the key factors, some oversimplification is unavoidable. But
I do acknowledge this limitation. I hope to improve things in the future.

With this, I have given you most of the key facts (except for a final piece of consideration described in Sections 9.5–9.8, that would help explain the qualitative
nature of subjective experiences afforded by mammalian brains). Together they
form an overall landscape on which a theory can be built. The readers who are
skeptical of others' theoretical speculations may take these facts for their own
purposes. In Chapter 7 we will introduce a theory. This view is a "centrist" position because it relates consciousness to broader notions of rational cognition
(Chapter 8), and at the same time it also addresses the philosophical problems of
"qualia," especially the biopsychic intuitions (Chapter 9).

References

Aitchison L, Lengyel M. With or without you: Predictive coding and Bayesian inference in the brain. *Curr Opin Neurobiol* 2017;**46**:219–227.

Block N. Inverted Earth. *Philos Perspect* 1990;**4**:53–79.

Braun AR, Balkin TJ, Wesensten NJ et al. Dissociated pattern of activity in visual
cortices and their projections during human rapid eye movement sleep. *Science*
1998;**279**:91–95.

Bridge H, Harrold S, Holmes EA et al. Vivid visual mental imagery in the absence of the primary visual cortex. *J Neurol* 2012;**259**:1062–1070.

Brown R. The brain and its states. In: S Edelman, T Fekete, N Zach (eds), *Being in Time: Dynamical Models of Phenomenal Experience*. 2012, John Benjamins, 211–230.

Brown R, Lau H, LeDoux JE. Understanding the higher-order approach to consciousness. *Trends Cogn Sci* 2019;**23**:754–768.

Cao R. New labels for old ideas: Predictive processing and the interpretation of neural signals. *Rev Philos Psychol* 2020;**11**:517–546.

Chalmers DJ. *The Conscious Mind: In Search of a Fundamental Theory*. Oxford Paperbacks, 1996.

Chang R, Baria AT, Flounders MW et al. Unconsciously elicited perceptual prior. *Neurosci Conscious* 2016;**2016**. https://doi.org/10.1093/nc/niw008.

Cleeremans A, Achoui D, Beauny A et al. Learning to be conscious. *Trends Cogn Sci* 2020;**24**:112–123.

Cortese A, Amano K, Koizumi A et al. Multivoxel neurofeedback selectively modulates confidence without changing perceptual performance. *Nat Commun* 2016;7:13669.

Cowey A. The blindsight saga. *Exp Brain Res* 2010;**200**:3–24.

Dehaene S, Lau H, Kouider S. What is consciousness, and could machines have it? *Science* 2017;**358**:486–492.

Fleming SM. Awareness as inference in a higher-order state space. *Neurosci Conscious* 2020;**2020**:niz020.

Gershman SJ. The generative adversarial brain. Front. Artif. Intel. *Appl* 2019;2:18.

Gibson JJ. *The Senses Considered as Perceptual Systems* [With illustrations]. L Carmichael (ed). Boston: Houghton Mifflin, 1968.

Godfrey-Smith P. Mind, matter, and metabolism. *J Philos* 2016;**113**:481–506.

Goodfellow I, Bengio Y, Courville A. *Deep Learning*. MIT Press, 2016.

Harrison SA, Tong F. Decoding reveals the contents of visual working memory in early visual areas. *Nature* 2009;**458**:632–635.

Huang L, Wang L, Shen W et al. A source for awareness-dependent figure-ground segregation in human prefrontal cortex. *Proc Natl Acad Sci U S A* 2020;**117**:30836–30847.

Hupé JM, James AC, Girard P et al. Response modulations by static texture surround in area V1 of the macaque monkey do not depend on feedback connections from V2. *J Neurophysiol* 2001;**85**:146–163.

Iijima K, Sakai KL. Subliminal enhancement of predictive effects during syntactic processing in the left inferior frontal gyrus: An MEG study. *Front Syst Neurosci* 2014;**8**:217.

Lau H. Consciousness, metacognition, & perceptual reality monitoring. 2019. Preprint. https://doi.org/10.31234/osf.io/ckbyf.

Lau H, Brown R. The emperor's new phenomenology? The empirical case for conscious experiences without first-order representations. In: A Pautz, D Stoljar (eds), *Blockheads! Essays on Ned Block's Philosophy of Mind and Consciousness*. MIT Press, 2019, 171.

Lau HC, Passingham RE. Relative blindsight in normal observers and the neural correlate of visual consciousness. *Proc Natl Acad Sci U S A* 2006;**103**:18763–18768.

LeDoux JE, Brown R. A higher-order theory of emotional consciousness. *Proc Natl Acad Sci U S A* 2017;**114**:E2016–E2025.

LeDoux JE, Michel M, Lau H. A little history goes a long way toward understanding why we study consciousness the way we do today. *Proc Natl Acad Sci U S A* 2020;**117**:6976–6984.

Maniscalco B, Lau H. The signal processing architecture underlying subjective reports of sensory awareness. *Neurosci Conscious* 2016;**2016**. https://doi.org/10.1093/nc/niw002.

Maniscalco B, Peters MAK, Lau H. Heuristic use of perceptual evidence leads to dissociation between performance and metacognitive sensitivity. *Atten Percept Psychophys* 2016;**78**:923–937.

Manita S, Suzuki T, Homma C et al. A top-down cortical circuit for accurate sensory perception. *Neuron* 2015;**86**:1304–1316.

Meijs EL, Slagter HA, de Lange FP et al. Dynamic interactions between top–down expectations and conscious awareness. *J Neurosci* 2018;**38**:2318–2327.

Mendoza-Halliday D, Martinez-Trujillo JC. Neuronal population coding of perceived and memorized visual features in the lateral prefrontal cortex. *Nat Commun* 2017;**8**:15471.

Michel M, Lau H. Is blindsight possible under signal detection theory? Comment on Phillips (2021). *Psychol Rev* 2021;**128**:585–591.

Miyoshi K, Lau H. A decision-congruent heuristic gives superior metacognitive sensitivity under realistic variance assumptions. *Psychol Rev* 2020;**127**:655–671.

Nourski KV, Steinschneider M, Rhone AE et al. Auditory predictive coding across awareness states under anesthesia: An intracranial electrophysiology study. *J Neurosci* 2018;**38**:8441–8452.

Parras GG, Nieto-Diego J, Carbajal GV et al. Neurons along the auditory pathway exhibit a hierarchical organization of prediction error. *Nat Commun* 2017;**8**:2148.

Peters MAK, Fesi J, Amendi N et al. Transcranial magnetic stimulation to visual cortex induces suboptimal introspection. *Cortex* 2017a;**93**:119–132.

Peters MAK, Kentridge RW, Phillips I et al. Does unconscious perception really exist? Continuing the ASSC20 debate. *Neurosci Conscious* 2017b;**2017**:nix015.

Peters MAK, Thesen T, Ko YD et al. Perceptual confidence neglects decision-incongruent evidence in the brain. *Nat Hum Behav* 2017c;**1**. https://doi.org/10.1038/s41562-017-0139.

Phillips I. Blindsight is qualitatively degraded conscious vision. *Psychol Rev* 2020.128;3;558–584. https://doi.org/10.1037/rev0000254.

Roelofs L. *Combining Minds: How to Think About Composite Subjectivity*. Oxford University Press, 2019.

Rosenthal, D. Consciousness and mind. Clarendon Press, 2005..

Rowe EG, Tsuchiya N, Garrido MI. Detecting (un)seen change: The neural underpinnings of (un)conscious prediction errors. *Front Syst Neurosci* 2020;14:81.

Zeman A, Dewar M, Della Sala S. Lives without imagery: Congenital aphantasia. *Cortex* 2015;73:378–380.

7

Are We Alone?

7.1 The Need for a Theory

In the introduction to this volume we cautioned against radical theorizing. As a discipline, we probably enjoy inventing new theories too much. Theoretical novelty has become too much of a good thing.

But theories are needed sometimes. As we address the remaining issues of consciousness in animals and robots, direct empirical evidence can only go so far. Some may feel that certain animals are capable of behavior so complex and human-like that it seems absurd to deny that they are conscious. But what if a robot can mimic these exact same behaviors? Is it then conscious too? Not infrequently, the reaction is much more skeptical in that case. We seem to lack a coherent set of objective criteria for making these judgments.

A good way to address this may be to first figure out what *in principle* accounts for consciousness in the human cases. From there, we can see if similar mechanisms exist or not in the animals or robots. This will provide no deductive proof, of course. It assumes that our knowledge of consciousness in humans is correct, *and* that the principles generalize to other creatures. But this is still far better than subjective guesses. To make this inductive generalization, we need a theory of consciousness.

Because neither the global nor local views work well, we need a third option. The theory doesn't have to be brand new; it is more important that it is correct. In the chapter I'll introduce what can be considered a variant of a higher-order theory (Lau and Rosenthal 2011), which I call the perceptual reality monitoring (PRM) theory (Lau 2019). The key ideas can be traced back to John Locke and Immanuel Kant, among others. As I mentioned in Chapter 6, David Rosenthal and Richard Brown are two contemporary champions of variants of this philosophical theory. Rather than proposing something radically new, I will express similar ideas in different terms. But I'll also point out some key differences between our views in Sections 7.4–7.6. The goal is not to contrive originality. Rather, it is to defend that these ideas are generally empirically plausible, and very much compatible with the scientific evidence reviewed in earlier chapters.

In Consciousness We Trust. Hakwan Lau, Oxford University Press. © Hakwan Lau 2022.
DOI: 10.1093/oso/9780198856771.003.0008

7.2 Some Intuitions

On the internet, there are videos of various animals reacting to magic tricks. In one of my favorite demonstrations, a person presented a simple trick to an orangutan. The person placed an object inside a cup, shook it, and then removed the object quickly with a sleight of hand. Afterwards, when the orangutan looked into the cup and couldn't find the object, the animal looked puzzled for a second, and then rolled on the floor with what seemed like bewildered amusement.

Let us assume that we read the emotion of the animal correctly: that the animal was in fact entertained. Can we imagine this animal not having conscious vision? That is, could the animal just be sensing visual information effectively, without having subjective experiences? Perhaps it was something equivalent to a very powerful form of blindsight?

But a blindsight patient may not find magic tricks so entertaining either. Let's say a patient can track the permanence of a moving object, so "guesses" can be made correctly as to whether an object suddenly disappears. Would the patient find this so amazing to watch? Perhaps it is possible the patient may have a gut reaction that something funny is going on when an object suddenly disappears. But to enjoy stage magic involves more than that. When we go to magic shows we hope not just to be nonconsciously "tickled." When we find a magic trick amazing, we enjoy the sense of amazement *as a rational agent*. We find it entertaining in large part because these tricks challenge our grasp of reality. Things appear *crazy*!

So there may be an argument to be made, that there is really no such thing as nonconscious magic tricks. The "unbelievable" nature of magic tricks is a major source of the amusement. But this conflict between our perception and beliefs seems to arise only for conscious perception. In blindsight, the nonconscious perceptual information is in a sense cognitively accessible too, as reflected by the guessing behavior. But the information does not impinge on the patients' belief system the same way as conscious perception does. Blindsight patients don't automatically form firm and rational beliefs when they nonconsciously encounter objects in the world.

Perhaps this lack of direct connection to our beliefs is not specific to blindsight, but true for nonconscious perception in general. If that is so, this may explain why some of us find it so difficult to see how the orangutan could have seen the magic trick only nonconsciously. If the animal lacked conscious vision, the trick just wouldn't have been so genuinely interesting.

7.3 Optimal Bayesians & Phantom Pain

Intuitions are not universal. Unlike me, others may not find it so hard to imagine that a nonconscious animal can somehow enjoy magic tricks too. Or
maybe there could be a form of super-blindsight, in which subjective experience is lacking and yet it can directly lead to very *firm* beliefs.

But this firmness of perceptual beliefs deserves further consideration. They
say seeing is believing. But as far as conscious seeing is concerned, the result
is typically not just some ordinary, casual beliefs, like believing that tomorrow
is going to rain. We believe what we consciously see with a certain degree of
conviction and immediacy. In most cases, it feels like it is the most reasonable thing to hold on to these beliefs—sometimes even in the face of contradictory evidence. Philosophers sometimes say that perception comes with an
"assertoric force." It tells us about what is going on *here and now*, in ways that
we can't quite ignore.

This seems to go against the general wisdom for building a rational decision-
making system. Engineers and cognitive theorists who take probability theory
seriously sometimes identify themselves as Bayesians (after Thomas Bayes's
famous theorem on conditional probabilities). These scholars recognize that
evidence comes with varying degrees of strength. The optimal way to make
decisions is to combine *all* of the different sources of evidence, as weighted by
their respective reliability. This is to say, in the face of contradictory evidence,
no single source should by default dominate in absolute terms. Let's say I am
very sure that today is Monday. But if all my friends tell me that today actually
is Tuesday, instead, I will probably check the calendar on the internet. If it is
confirmed that they are correct, I will revise my belief. I should let the new information override my former conviction and conclude that I was mistaken.
The former belief would not retain some mysterious "assertoric force."

Curiously, with conscious perception, this assertoric force seems to never
go away. Take the example of phantom pain, which happens in some patients
with amputated limbs (Nikolajsen et al. 1997). These patients may feel pain
in the limbs that they no longer have. Yet these patients are typically perfectly
rational and lucid. They know about the amputation, and the impossibility
to have a bodily disturbance in the "location" of the pain per se. And yet they
can't *reason* the pain away. They cannot just take into account other evidence
and beliefs and let them override and eliminate the "mistaken" pain. The subjective experience remains, and so does the assertoric force. It continues to
feel *as if* something is wrong (e.g., being stabbed at) in the location where the
pain is felt.

So this assertoric force seems strangely *stubborn*, in the way it has this tendency to inform us about what's happening *here and now*, regardless of what background beliefs we have. With effort we can resist believing in what we currently see, but things would still *seem* to us a certain way, given our conscious percepts. If we are anything like an optimal Bayesian system, the process of evidence accumulation is really not supposed to work this way. As such, perhaps we shouldn't expect nonconscious perception to ever behave like this either. This assertoric force may be a unique and curious feature of consciousness that calls for an explanation.

7.4 Higher-Order Thought or Beliefs?

One way to account for the assertoric force discussed in Section 7.3 is to theorize that conscious perception always involves two sets of representations. We can call the state of early sensory activity the first-order state or first-order representation. This reflects the perceptual content (e.g., what objects are involved and in what spatial location, with specific features like colors, size, and motion direct). These representations are likely within the sensory cortices. We can say they are relatively picture-like, carrying analog content; we will discuss more what "analog" means in Section 9.5.

However, for one to consciously perceive, one may additionally need to have certain higher-order states or representations. That is, the first-order states alone may drive visual behavior and performance. But without the relevant higher-order states, that would only constitute nonconscious perception, as in blindsight. The higher-order states may be reflected by activity in, for example, the prefrontal cortex. The content of these representations may be more conceptual, symbolic, and relatively sentence-like.

What may be the specific content of the higher-order states? Given the discussion in the Section 7.3, one may be tempted to think that these higher-order states could be the corresponding perceptual beliefs. That is, the first-order state contains the picture-like sensory information, for example, about a cat in front of us. For us to consciously see the cat, we need to have the higher-order belief *that* there is the cat in front of us. This belief can then guide our rational decision-making.

But this higher-order "belief" view is too strong. What conscious perception entails is an assertoric force. But this force does not *always* lead to the corresponding belief. For example, some individuals knowingly ingest hallucinogens for recreational purposes. When they hallucinate a cat, they don't necessarily believe that a cat is really out there in front of them. That is, their background beliefs may ultimately override the assertoric force given by conscious perception. Likewise for the phantom pain example from the last section. Those patients typically don't end up believing that there is bodily disturbance in the location of the felt pain. It just feels *as if* there is such bodily disturbance there. But they know full well that this is impossible in reality because the relevant limb no longer exists.

So what we want is for conscious perception to have the strong *tendency*, but not logical necessity, to lead to the corresponding perceptual belief. Some philosophers have argued for such a "dispositionalist" position (Pitcher 1971). But just stating that there is such a strong disposition doesn't quite make a scientific theory. We need some account of how that disposition comes about.

One influential view is David Rosenthal's higher-order thought theory (2005), which may be an attractive candidate solution here. Continuing with the example of having a first-order representation of a cat, the corresponding higher-order "thought" may have content like: I am having a first-order representation of a cat. Because of this thought, one can account for why one may be disposed to making the corresponding belief; in the absence of contradictory background beliefs, the relevant perceptual belief logically follows.

But if that is the relevant higher-order content, we face another kind of problem. In Section 6.10 we mentioned that the sensory representations may be similar whether it is externally triggered or endogenously generated. These representations are not exactly identical, but seeing a cat and maintaining the image of it in working memory both involve having a first-order representation of a cat. And yet, the mere thought that one is in such a first-order state does not always lead to subjective visual experience. The phenomenology of visual working memory varies across individuals. Some people do not experience imagery during memory delay at all (Zeman, Dewar, and Della Sala 2015). And yet they are no doubt aware of holding the content in mind; they *think* they are in the relevant first-order state—even though there is no corresponding visual experience. Even for those who experience vivid imagery during working-memory delays, the experience is different from normal perception. It lacks that *here and now* quality.

Perhaps this reading of Rosenthal's higher-order thought theory is not so charitable. Maybe the relevant higher-order thought could be more specific: for example, I am seeing a cat *versus* I am holding the image of a cat in working memory. This way we can stipulate that only the former leads to the subjective experience of seeing but the latter doesn't. But the requirements for a philosophical theory may be different from what we need for a scientific theory. Given our purpose here, we should have a mechanistic explanation for how these different higher-order states come about. Just saying that these may be the possible contents in abstract terms isn't very satisfying. Ideally, we should be able to describe them in enough detail so that we can in principle *build* a system capable of generating these higher-order states.

7.5　Inner Sense

In Section 6.10, we introduced generative adversarial networks (GANs). To facilitate the development of a system capable of predictive coding, a "discriminator" may be employed. The job of this discriminator is exactly to distinguish between the different kinds of first-order states described in the last section: endogenously generated versus externally triggered. So we can think of the discriminator as a higher-order mechanism for consciousness.

One interesting feature of the discriminator is that it is basically just a simple *perceptual* categorization network. In this sense the higher-order process itself isn't exactly thought—or sentence-like (although it may output to further downstream processes that are more so). So, this may correspond to another variant of higher-order theory known as "inner-sense" theory, or higher-order *perception* theories. These theories have been criticized on philosophical grounds (Carruthers 2007), but I'm not sure the arguments are decisive.

In particular, one challenge raised by critics of the "inner-sense" theory is empirical (Sauret and Lycan 2014). They argued that no such inner-sense "organ" has been found. But today we know that there may be good computational reasons why the brain would have employed a GANs-like architecture. The neurophysiological evidence suggests that such a mechanism may be in the prefrontal cortex (Section 6.10). And then computationally, it seems like the same mechanism could be repurposed for metacognition. This in turn neatly explains why disrupting activity in the prefrontal cortex, where such discriminator function likely locates, can impair metacognition too (Chapter 3).

I mentioned the above "repurposing" finding as a result of a computational modeling exercise (Section 6.10). But conceptually we can also understand why the discriminator may be useful for metacognition. In general, if one becomes very good at distinguishing between two subtypes of X, one tends also to be better at detecting X from non-X. For example, if we are really good at telling red wines from white wines by taste, chances are we can detect just in a sip if some wine has been added to a glass of water too. So likewise, since the discriminator is capable of distinguishing between internally generated and externally triggered first-order states, it makes sense that it can distinguish the presence of a perceptual signal from sheer noise too.

This metacognitive function—of distinguishing between a meaningful perceptual signal and noise—is important because spontaneous neuronal activity is ubiquitous. It accounts for much of the metabolic budget of the brain (Raichle 2006; Schölvinck, Howarth, and Attwell 2008). As I'm writing, my cat-representing neurons, like most other sensory neurons, fire now and then. But I do not hallucinate seeing cats (!). Somewhere there must be a mechanism in the brain for deciding that such spontaneous activity is just "noise," rather than caused by a cat in front of me.

Let's assume that an agent is capable of reasoning with beliefs and goals. If the mechanisms for this kind of general symbolic-level cognition receive input from both the first-order states and the discriminator, one can see how conscious perception can attain its assertoric force. Essentially, conscious perception happens when the first-order state represents the cat, *and* the higher-order (discriminator) state indicates that the first-order state is a true reflection of the world right now. Together, these two representations constitute something akin to the premises of a syllogistic inference. In the absence of conflicting background beliefs, it is rational to form the belief that there is a cat in front of us right now. Such a belief is in a sense "justified" by the premises; it logically follows (Figure 7.1).

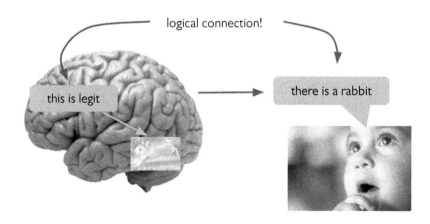

Figure 7.1 Perceptual reality monitoring via first- and higher-order representations

7.6 Index, Gating, & the Richness of Experience

The last point sets the theory apart from most other versions of higher-order theories because here perceptual beliefs are derived from both the first-order (sensory) and higher-order (discriminator) states. In higher-order thought theory, the content of consciousness is ultimately determined by the higher-order state (Rosenthal 2005; Lau and Brown 2019). The first-order state is the normal cause or input to the higher-order state, but it isn't constitutively part of the subjective experience. Once the higher-order state is formed, in principle, both the subjective experience and the relevant perceptual beliefs can occur with or without the first-order state.

Against the higher-order thought view, there may be some concerns regarding whether the thought-like higher-order representation can capture the richness of perceptual experience. As reviewed in Chapter 4, the issue is controversial. But a standard higher-order *thought* theorist is committed to a relatively "sparse" view, on which perceptual experience is no richer than what can be captured by conceptual, thought-like representations. The view argued for here makes no such commitment; the rich content of the first-order state also contributes. The higher-order state does not duplicate the first-order content, but merely serves as a gating mechanism to direct the first-order information to the relevant downstream processes.

The reader may wonder: how does the higher-order (discriminator) state *refer* to the corresponding first-order state, without duplicating its content? In current artificial GANs, we tend to deal with just one first-order state at a time. But in the actual human brain, there may be multiple concurrent perceptual states in different sensory modalities. At a given time, some of these first-order states may lead to subjective experience while others may not. As such, there are likely multiple discriminator outputs, and one needs to keep track of which refers to which first-order states. Of relevance is that *indexing* or variable binding mechanisms have been proposed for prefrontal functions (Kriete et al. 2013). Essentially, the prefrontal cortex must have some ways of referring to specific first-order activities via some form of "addressing" system.

For a simplistic analogy, we can think of this as a phone numbers system, where each individual referent is given a unique identifier. So, as in modern computational systems, a higher-order mechanism can refer to first-order representations by these addresses, without duplicating or redescribing the full content. In Chapter 9 we will revisit how such mechanisms may actually work in the mammalian sensory cortices.

For these indexes or addresses to work, they need to be interpretable by some downstream system. Such a system must be able to access both the higher-order and first-order content. On the view advocated here, the idea is that these contents are subsequently read out by the mechanisms for general symbolic-level cognition and logical reasoning. In this sense, consciousness is the *gating mechanism* by which perception impacts cognition; it selects what perceptual information should directly influence our rational thinking.

Note that this is not to identify consciousness with access consciousness (as discussed in Section 1.6). *Consciousness* here refers to subjective experience, as we do throughout most of this book. The point is that subjective experiences are *causally* connected with access consciousness in the ways described above. Subjective experiences are characterized by their *availability* for *potential* conscious access. But I'm not suggesting that the two are one and the same. When the discriminator decides that a first-order representation correctly represents the world right now, global broadcast and access are *likely* to happen. But these consequences are not constitutively part of the subjective experience, according to this view.

7.7 Phenomenology of Imagery

We can call the view introduced in the last few sections the PRM theory. It is so-called because in the memory literature, a similar process of reality monitoring has been proposed (Johnson and Raye 1981; Johnson 1988). For example, young children and older adults alike sometimes confuse their own past imagination with events that actually took place. This could lead to dire consequences, if they were in fact mistaken and to bear witness in court cases, for example. Fortunately, this doesn't happen more often, because monitoring mechanisms exist in the brain to determine the source of a memory. This allows us to tell apart reality from fantasy, in a generally reliable fashion. By identifying such reality monitoring mechanisms in the prefrontal cortex (Simons, Garrison, and Johnson 2017), we can also in principle assess how trustworthy one's witness statements may be, based on neurological data.

Likewise, in the case of perceptual signals, there is a similar need to distinguish between reality and our own mental imagery. But does PRM imply that endogenously generated perceptual signals are always nonconscious? The short answer is *no*. But it is somewhat complicated.

What is clear is that normal functioning subjects do not generally confuse normal perception with imagery; the phenomenology is typically distinct in the two cases. There has been some scant evidence that such confusion is common, but the results, at least in their original forms, are not robustly replicable (Segal and Nathan 1964; Segal and Gordon 1969). Modern empirical studies have found relatively subtle interference between perception and endogenously maintained perceptual information (Kang et al. 2011; Salahub and Emrich 2016; Teng and Kravitz 2019; Dijkstra and Fleming 2021; Dijkstra et al. 2021; Dijkstra, Kok, and Fleming 2021).

But what is the phenomenology for endogenously generated perceptual signals? Is it distinct from normal perception because it is "weaker" or absent? There are considerable individual differences regarding the phenomenology of mental imagery. In aphantasia, the concerned individuals do not experience visual imagery in vivid forms at all (Zeman, Dewar, and Della Sala 2015). One possibility is that the relevant first-order sensory states are either absent or only partially instantiated when these subjects engage in visual thinking. But how come one can still perform visual functions without these first-order activities?

According to PRM, there is another possibility why aphantasia or weak imagery experience may happen. We have argued that the neural mechanisms for the discriminator may also contribute to metacognition. So in total, this discriminator-like mechanism has *three* different output conditions. That is, a first-order state is one of the following: i) externally triggered, ii) internally generated, or iii) just noise. The first condition should lead to normal subjective perceptual experience, and that the third condition should entail the lack of subjective experience. When the discriminator decides that a certain first-order state is internally generated (second condition), a distinct output is needed. Whether this output is more similar to the first or the third condition may vary across people; when we say two outputs are similar, we mean that they are more easily confused to be the same by downstream readout. To the extent that it is more similar to the third condition (noise) rather than the first (externally triggered), PRM predicts that subjective experience may be absent or relatively feeble too—even if the first-order activity is actually robust.

Incidentally, although neurophysiological and anatomical correlates of imagery vividness have been found in sensory areas, similar findings have also been reported for prefrontal and parietal areas (Dijkstra, Bosch, and van Gerven 2019). The relative paucity of evidence for the higher-order areas may again be due to methodological considerations already discussed in Chapters 2 and 3. As such, one may hypothesize that imagery vividness can be causally manipulated if we tamper with *either* the first-order or the higher-order states (appropriately). I am not aware of this being formally tested yet: to induce confusion between imagery and perception with prefrontal or parietal stimulations. PRM hereby makes this empirical prediction.

7.8 Implicit Versus Explicit Reality Monitoring: The Case of Dreams

The last point highlights why PRM is a balanced synthesis between local and global theories. Local theorists emphasize the causal relevance of early sensory mechanisms. They certainly have a point, but that picture is empirically incomplete. In reaction, global theorists sometimes come across as putting too much emphasis on the prefrontal and parietal cortices alone. But both the higher-order and first-order states are important. Various "disorders" of consciousness can be caused by abnormalities in either (Zmigrod et al. 2016). A correct theory must be able to account for both.

The common phenomenon of dreaming is typically not considered a "disorder." But in dreams we are typically "mistaken" in a sense: we treat our internally generated sensory activities as reflecting the present state of the world. In other words, dreams are a form of hallucinations. As in other kinds of hallucinations, there are no doubt first-order correlates (i.e., activities in the sensory regions of the brain; Horikawa et al. 2013). But as we have pointed out, working memory and mental imagery also involve similar early sensory activities. And yet in dreams the sensations seem far more vivid. One may argue that during working memory and mental imagery the sensory activities are perhaps not as strong and detailed. But in dreams these activities are also generated endogenously. In all these cases, concurrent external input is lacking. What sets the corresponding subjective experiences apart?

Although not all dreams happen during REM (rapid eye movements) sleep, we dream more often during REM than non-REM sleep. Incidentally, during REM sleep sensory cortices tend to be active, and yet prefrontal areas like the dorsolateral prefrontal cortex often show reduced levels of activity (Muzur, Pace-Schott, and Hobson 2002). This has been taken as a challenge to traditional versions of the higher-order view; perhaps less activity in the prefrontal cortex means fewer higher-order thoughts, and those one should not be having vivid experiences as we do in dreams. But as we explained in Chapter 3, neurons in the prefrontal cortex do not fire to signal simply the presence of a stimulus. Instead, they form complex high-dimensional neuronal population codes. As such, we need to be careful in interpreting the lack of salient prefrontal activity as observed by crude neuroimaging measures during REM sleep. One plausible interpretation is that during REM sleep the prefrontal areas may be *failing* their usual role in PRM, leading us to mistake endogenously generated sensory activities as caused directly by the external world. The low activity exactly reflects the disengagement of the relevant process.

Incidentally, we are not always mistaken about the nature of dreams. Occasionally, people have lucid dreams, in which they know full well that they are dreaming. They know that their subjective experiences are detached from reality. Lucid dreaming has been associated with heightened activity in the prefrontal cortex (Dresler et al. 2012; Stumbrys, Erlacher, and Schredl 2013). Perhaps this is why we recognize the illusory nature of dream percepts during lucid dreams.

However, an important distinction needs to be made. In lucid dreams we continue to have vivid subjective experiences. The correct and explicit monitoring of reality happens at a higher cognitive level. This is similar to the case of known hallucinations described in Section 7.4. Even if we don't ultimately form the mistaken beliefs, the subjective experiences in dreams and known hallucinations are still somewhat misleading, as they carry this undeserved "assertoric force." So for these instances, we can say that reality monitoring fails at this implicit, subpersonal, and automatic level, even though this is corrected downstream at the higher cognitive, explicit level.

For PRM and subjective experience, it is this *implicit* kind of reality monitoring that really matters. The idea is that the prefrontal cortex may be important for *both* kinds of reality monitoring, implicit (i.e., subpersonal) as well as explicit (i.e., higher cognitive). If one fails, the other may not; the relevant circuits need not be exactly identical, even though they may partially overlap, and may both reside within the prefrontal cortex. The partial overlap between the explicit and implicit functions may explain why lucid dreaming is possible but relatively rare; it requires the explicit reality monitoring to function but implicit reality monitoring to fail.

There is some evidence in support for the idea that the prefrontal cortex may be important for both kinds of metacognition in dreams, explicit and implicit, although the mechanisms may be ultimately different. Applying transcranial electrical stimulation through the scalp, Voss et al (2014) have reported that targeting the prefrontal cortex can increase incidents of lucid dreaming (explicit metacognition). However, such stimulation also seems to have effects on the reported frequency of dreams, as well as the reported degree of "realism" of the sensory details in dream content (see the supplementary tables in Voss et al. 2014). Subjects seem to more frequently mistake endogenously generated "noise" as reflecting the outside world (*failure* of implicit metacognition).

Based on electroencephalogram (EEG) data, others have suggested that some regions in the medial parietal areas may be important for subjective experiences to arise in dreams too (Siclari et al. 2017). This is not in contradiction with higher-order theories; although the prefrontal cortex is often emphasized, both global and higher-order theorists actually also recognize the importance of other areas in the association cortices, including parietal areas (see Section 3.1). But one concern is that some of these areas, such as the precuneus, are also linked to memory metacognition (as reviewed in Chapter 3) and the vividness of memory recall (Richter et al. 2016). So one needs to make sure the activity truly reflects subjective experience *per se*, rather than just the memory and subsequent reportability of these experiences.

One should also note that in the EEG study mentioned above, prefrontal activities were also found for subsequently reported dreams (Siclari et al. 2017). The researcher wrote off such activity as relatively weak and inconsistent. But as in the findings on REM sleep mentioned above, such weak signals may actually reflect the failure of subpersonal PRM, which can be the causal explanation for subjective experiences in dreams. Also, with a relatively crude method like EEG we should not overinterpret null or weak results. Imaging methods do not give the same sensitivity to different signals in different regions, as we have already discussed in Chapter 3. Fazekas and Nemeth (2018) provide a useful review suggesting that the emphasis on medial parietal areas at the expense of prefrontal involvement may be empirically unsound.

7.9 Other Higher-Order Failures

Why do we think that both explicit and implicit PRM depend on the same brain regions? I take it that for the explicit, higher-cognitive variant, it is not controversial that the prefrontal cortex is important. Failure of reality monitoring at this level amounts to general delusions. The prefrontal cortex is known to be important for normal cognitive functioning and reasoning.

But just because explicit metacognition and explicit PRM depend on the prefrontal cortex does not mean that the relevant implicit processes must be carried out in earlier sensory regions. A single cortical area often subserves multiple functions. Given the similarity in the overall computational goal, it would make sense that the implicit and explicit circuits are in close proximity or may partially overlap. Assuming explicit metacognition and reality monitoring are evolutionarily "newer" functions, they may be built upon the relevant implicit mechanisms, "recycling" some of the same neural resources and similar circuits. But it does not mean that the explicit and implicit functions are the same.

Phil Corlett has made the argument that higher-cognitive delusions and sensory hallucinations may not be driven by totally independent factors, as they sometimes suggested (2019). Many current theories of psychosis identify dopaminergic functions in the prefrontal cortex as key mechanistic components (Braver, Barch, and Cohen 1999). Again, this is not to say that when patients with schizophrenia hallucinate, early sensory activities are irrelevant. The point is that perhaps the higher-order mechanisms in the prefrontal cortex are important too, even in the absence of delusions. The prefrontal cortex may be the common factor in *both* sensory-level hallucinations as well as higher-cognitive delusions. We will address further in Chapter 8 how malfunctions at the two levels may interact.

An often overlooked fact is that some patients with Parkinson's disease or Lewy body dementia also hallucinate visually (Onofrj et al. 2013). Unlike patients with schizophrenia, they are relatively lucid and cognitively intact. Again, Parkinson's disease is characterized by impairments of dopaminergic functions in the frontal lobes, including the subcortical basal ganglia (Narayanan, Rodnitzky, and Uc 2013).

Finally, as we already discussed in Chapter 2 Section 2.11, even for a disorder of subjective experience caused by lesion to the primary visual cortex—blindsight—there are clear physiological correlates in the prefrontal cortex. Theoretically it has been suggested that higher-order malfunctioning is the ultimate culprit (Ko and Lau 2012).

7.10 Inflation Revisited

Section 7.9 may help us understand the possible role of prefrontal mechanisms in inflation. Recall from Chapter 4 that *inflation* refers to the occurrence of subjective experience under the relative lack of representational details. This may happen in peripheral vision, for instance.

Suppose we have the first-order sensory state of a cat that is rather impoverished. As a pictorial representation it lacks details. The content barely reflects a real cat. There is no way to tell if it is a Persian cat or a Bengal, or neither. So, an unbiased optimal system may well consider this to be noise, rather than a truthful representation of the current state of the world. The representation just isn't reliable enough to be taken seriously.

But according to PRM, the relevant higher-order mechanism is distinct from the first-order state. If the higher-order mechanism *somehow* makes the judgment that the impoverished first-order state correctly reflects the current world, according to the theory there will be a corresponding subjective experience. Instead of being filtered out from further processing, the weak first-order representation would be available for higher-cognitive access. There will be an assertoric force that comes with the conscious experience, to the effect that "something like a cat" (or whatever represented by the first-order state) is in front of the subject. This may explain why in peripheral or un-attended vision, there is a robust liberal detection bias, even when one is not so able to discriminate or identify the relevant target well (Section 4.9). The perceptual content ultimately lacks the detail, so upon reflection it may not be "rich" per se. But if it is being deemed by the higher-order mechanism as rich enough, there is a sense in which the perceptual experience is subjectively rich or strong; the subject is likely to form the corresponding belief with certainty.

Why would the higher-order mechanism make such a biased judgment, given that the first-order state isn't quite detailed and robust enough to be re-liably distinguished from noise? One reason is that the higher-order mech-anism may err, as we have discussed in the Sections 7.8 and 7.9. But such an "error" may also be a useful heuristic. For example, in peripheral or un-attended vision, the first-order state is *expected* to lack certain details. But that is not because *the world* lacks such details. Rather, our brains should "know" that such details are just a saccade away; we only have to look. So despite the lack of richness in the first-order content for the unattended periphery at one moment, the higher-order mechanism may reasonably give such content some "advanced" credit.

This account of inflation may apply also to the phenomenology of dreams. Although dreams feel vivid, upon reflection it is often unclear if all the details are really there. Perhaps it only *feels as if* the rich details are there—just as in peripheral or unattended vision.

7.11 Agency & Emotions

Although much of the evidence and analysis come from vision, PRM is meant to apply to all sensory modalities. But what about other experiences such as volition and emotions?

One could envision something like this: like perceptual representations, representations for action in the motor cortex are also activated in different ways (Gallese and Goldman 1998; Oosterhof, Tipper, and Downing 2012; Taube et al. 2015; Zabicki et al. 2017). When one imagines acting a certain way, there are similar neural activities as if one is performing the same action. When one observes another person making the action, similar activities also arise. And of course, spontaneous neural activity is ubiquitous. So there is a need for volitional reality monitoring too.

Likewise for affective reality monitoring: experiencing an emotion seems to activate some similar neural activities as when one is merely imagining it, or thinking about another person experiencing it (Sato et al. 2004; Singer et al.

2004). And of course neurons in affect-related brain regions such as the amygdala and insular also show spontaneous neural activity. So perhaps a similar discriminator or reality monitoring mechanisms may be at work in the prefrontal cortex.

But I suspect that there is more to it for the sense of agency and emotional experiences. These conscious experiences are in a sense more complex, as they involve a more explicit notion of the self (LeDoux and Lau 2020). Higher-cognitive and memory mechanisms may contribute to these experiences more than they do for simple perceptual experiences. We will address these possibilities further in Chapter 8.

7.12 Other Minds

With the above caveats in mind, we can finally address the question we started with in this chapter: besides us humans, what else is conscious? Specifically, let us set aside the potentially more complicated question regarding the sense of volitional control and emotions. What creatures are capable of having the simplest conscious perceptual experiences?

I started off with stage magic as an intuitive example. But of course that would not constitute a universally practical test for consciousness. One may need to be capable of having subjective perceptual experiences in order to appreciate stage magic, but other cognitive abilities may also be required.

To determine consciousness we need to get at the precise mechanisms. The relevant creature should first be capable of predictive coding, in a specific way. In particular, when the system generates sensory activity in a top-down manner, it should make use of the same machinery for bottom-up perception. This creates a need for a mechanism akin to a "discriminator" in GANs. This discriminator also has to be capable of metacognition (i.e., to distinguish meaningful sensory representations from noise). Finally, there needs to be a general reasoning and belief-formation system to which the discriminator signals.

This kind of sensory predictive coding mechanism seems present in many mammals. But when it comes to the discriminator function, it is far less clear. There is some evidence that rats are capable of some degree of metacognition, and the mechanisms may also depend on the prefrontal cortex (Stolyarova et al. 2019). But are these the same mechanisms for PRM? It is known that the rodent and primate prefrontal cortices are markedly different, in terms of basic anatomy (Schaeffer et al. 2020).

Related to this was the finding that some neurons can distinguish between perceptual and working-memory content (Mendoza-Halliday and Martinez-Trujillo 2017). These neurons are found in a prefrontal region known to be important for metacognition (i.e., the dorsolateral prefrontal cortex) in monkeys. So far, we lack direct evidence in smaller animals.

And are rats capable of reasoning with their beliefs and desires? Do they really have a general cognitive system for rational thoughts, like we have?

Despite these unresolved issues, I'm inclined to think that most mammals capable of sensory predictive processing and metacognition are probably having some simple conscious experiences. That leaves many smaller animals out. I do not feel certain about this but at least we can spell out the sources of this uncertainty, as I did above.

How about young children and babies? It has been shown that preverbal infants are capable of some degree of metacognition (Goupil and Kouider 2016, 2019; Goupil, Romand-Monnier, and Kouider 2016). As in the case of smaller animals, it is not entirely clear if they make use of the exact same mechanisms for PRM. But because of their developmental trajectory the case may be stronger here. Also, although young children aren't capable of sophisticated reasoning with counter-factual beliefs, they are probably capable of some rational thinking based on beliefs and desires. So according to PRM they are likely conscious too.

That is to say, although some details may be currently not fully proven, these are empirically addressable issues. Assuming PRM is right, we can look for whether human infants and other animals have the essential mechanisms. This is a method of induction. We are assuming that PRM is correct not only in the subjects we have tested. We are hoping it generalizes. But this may be the best that we can do.

The more interesting case may be robots. There we do not have the same uncertainty driven by the lack of empirical data. Many current neural network models are capable of predictive processing. But typically, the generative model projects its top-down outputs to a set of nodes distinct from those used for bottom-up perception (Pu et al. 2016). So they do not have the same pressure to avoid the confusion. That said, some current models are already more brain-like, with the same sensory circuits being used in both top-down and bottom-up processing (Rasmus et al. 2015). Also, of course, the very notion of the discriminator comes from neural network models.

The more challenging part may concern belief formation. Artificial General Intelligence, that is a computational system capable of human-like rational cognition, is a challenging goal (Goertzel 2014). While some current systems are capable of problem-solving and decision-making, it is not clear to what extent they resemble our cognitive architecture. In particular, it is unclear if such systems are truly capable of producing "thoughts" and "beliefs" in the general sense.

But at least in the current version of PRM, the commitment of the theory should be clear: to the extent a robot has such general reasoning capacities like we do, and if a discriminator signals to such mechanisms that a certain sensory representation is a truthful reflection of the current world, the robot will form a "conscious experience" of the relevant sensory content.

7.13 The Hard Enough Problem

The last point may sound so wild that some may see it as an exposition of the problem of the theory. A robot is just a machine. How can something as special as subjective experience come out of sheer computations?

I agree with this sentiment. Together with other authors I have previously speculated on the issue of machine consciousness (Dehaene, Lau, and Kouider 2017). But I have come to think that our proposal was unsatisfactory. Some key elements seem to be still missing. Perhaps in this preliminary version of PRM, it is not clear how the sense of self comes about, which may be important for at least some forms of conscious experiences (LeDoux and Lau 2020). In Chapter 8 we will try to address that.

But there is also a widespread intuition that the relevant substrate may also matter; this is what ultimately motivates biopsychism (as introduced in the Chapter 6). Machines made of electronics rather than wet, living brains, just seem incapable of *feeling what it is like* to be in certain subjective experiences. Maybe this is just an intuition. But I promise I will try to give my best shot at addressing this issue in the final chapter too.

For now, however, it is important for us to realize that this is a problem for all theories of consciousness. Once a mechanism of consciousness is spelled out, we can try to imagine building a simple creature just barely having the mechanism and proceed to consider if such a simple creature is plausibly conscious. Instead of fixating on the implausibility in absolute terms, we would do well to see how other theories fare and compare accordingly. We can call this the Hard Enough Problem. By "hard enough," I don't mean it is "pretty hard"; I mean that it is exactly hard *enough* for our purpose *of arbitrating between different theories*. The least implausible theory may be the best we can ever have.

Let us consider the robot described in Section 7.12 in more detail. It is true that it is not flesh and blood. But suppose it has some sensors for detecting bodily damage. When the discriminator tells its general reasoning system that the relevant sensory activity is correctly reflecting the world right now, it will form the belief that something in a certain part of the body is damaged. Suppose it is a false alarm; upon checking, that part of the body actually looks fine and functions well. But because of the way the discriminator is connected to the system for general cognition, it will continue to have this unshakable assertoric force, that something is wrong in that specific part of the body. It can't reason that signal away. That signal will continue to impinge on its rational thinking, *as if* that part of the body is damaged.

How different is this from pain as we know it?

But let us also consider similar cases for other theories of consciousness. For the global view, all it takes is the global broadcast of information, through some central information exchange system. Many current computer network systems already have such mechanisms. Are they conscious then?

And for the local theorist, if the right kind of local sensory activity is really all it takes, what if we isolate such activity so it does not make any downstream impact to other brain areas? What if we keep the relevant neurons in vitro, on a petri-dish, and stimulate them to mimic normal activity? Would they be conscious?

So, all current theories seem to make some rather improbable predictions. Of course, if we know *for sure* that a theory is correct, we should accept whatever improbable consequences it entails. But I hope the reader should have been convinced by now, that the science of consciousness is just no such simple matter. It would take some profound lack of critical thinking for one to accept that *any* current theory can be considered absolutely proven at the moment—including PRM, of course. So the Hard Enough Problem matters. And *perhaps* PRM offers one of the least implausible solutions for now.

If this doesn't feel quite plausible enough just yet, maybe something is in fact missing still. I hope that Chapter 8, and especially also Chapter 9, may convince you a bit more.

7.14 Chapter Summary

Consciousness in animals and robots is not an easy topic. Unfortunately, on this issue, scientists have often made premature and grandiose claims. These claims are rarely based on evidence and logic. Rather, philosophically unexamined intuitions masquerade as established scientific viewpoints. Here I try to make the case that this really should be a two-way process. First, we should see what the most empirically plausible theory says. Then in turn we should also evaluate the theory based on what the theory says about the matter. If it is just too outlandish, perhaps it would be grounds for rejecting the theory.

The theory I advocate, PRM, suggests that conscious experiences arise out of self-recognized perception of some sort. If a specific inner-sense mechanism "perceives" a sensory representation to be correctly reflecting the world at present, we become conscious of the sensory content. Because this mechanism directly impacts our rational thinking, consciousness can be understood as the *interface* between perception and cognition. Subjective experiences are the things that we are naturally inclined to believe—and *trust*.

PRM faces challenges from the Hard Enough Problem. Many may find it counter-intuitive that a robot can ever be conscious in the sense of having subjective, qualitative experiences. But the logic of the Hard Enough Problem is that it is a relative matter. It depends on what other theories say, which is often far more improbable.

So perhaps this is good enough. But some readers may feel that the theory still does not get at the qualitative aspect of *what it is like* to have a certain conscious experience. We will address this problem in Chapter 9, in order to finally give a better answer to the problem of machine consciousness. But before that, we need to first place the problem in a broader context, to see what really is at stake. In doing so, we will also expand the theory a bit in order to account for emotion and the subjective sense of agency, which are of course no less important than simple perceptual experiences.

References

Braver TS, Barch DM, Cohen JD. Cognition and control in schizophrenia: A computational model of dopamine and prefrontal function. *Biol Psychiatry* 1999;**46**:312–328.

Carruthers P. Higher-order theories of consciousness. *The Blackwell Companion to Consciousness*. Wiley-Blackwell Publishers, 2007;**10**:9780470751466.

Corlett PR. Factor one, familiarity and frontal cortex: A challenge to the two-factor theory of delusions. *Cogn Neuropsychiatry* 2019;**24**:165–177.

Dehaene S, Lau H, Kouider S. What is consciousness, and could machines have it? *Science* 2017;**358**:486–492.

Dijkstra N, Bosch SE, van Gerven MAJ. Shared neural mechanisms of visual perception and imagery. *Trends Cogn Sci* 2019;**23**:423–434.

Dijkstra N, Fleming SM. Fundamental constraints on distinguishing reality from imagination. 2021. https://doi.org/10.31234/osf.io/bw872.

Dijkstra N, Kok P, Fleming SM. Perceptual reality monitoring: Neural mechanisms dissociating imagination from reality. 2021. https://doi.org/10.31234/osf.io/zngeq.

Dijkstra N, Mazor M, Kok P et al. Mistaking imagination for reality: Congruent mental imagery leads to more liberal perceptual detection. *Cognition* 2021;**212**:104719.

Dresler M, Wehrle R, Spoormaker VI et al. Neural correlates of dream lucidity obtained from contrasting lucid versus non-lucid REM sleep: A combined EEG/fMRI case study. *Sleep* 2012;**35**:1017–1020.

Fazekas P, Nemeth G. Dream experiences and the neural correlates of perceptual consciousness and cognitive access. *Philos Trans R Soc Lond B Biol Sci* 2018;**373**. https://doi.org/10.1098/rstb.2017.0356.

Gallese V, Goldman A. Mirror neurons and the simulation theory of mind-reading. *Trends Cogn Sci* 1998;**2**:493–501.

Goertzel B. Artificial general intelligence: Concept, state of the art, and future prospects. *J Artif Gen Intell* 2014;**5**:1–48.

Goupil L, Kouider S. Behavioral and neural indices of metacognitive sensitivity in preverbal infants. *Curr Biol* 2016;**26**:3038–3045.

Goupil L, Kouider S. Developing a reflective mind: From core metacognition to explicit self-reflection. *Curr Dir Psychol Sci* 2019;**28**:403–408.

Goupil L, Romand-Monnier M, Kouider S. Infants ask for help when they know they don't know. *Proc Natl Acad Sci* 2016;**113**:3492–3496.

Horikawa T, Tamaki M, Miyawaki Y et al. Neural decoding of visual imagery during sleep. *Science* 2013;**340**:639–642.

Johnson MK. Reality monitoring: An experimental phenomenological approach. *J Exp Psychol Gen* 1988;**117**:390–394.

Johnson MK, Raye CL. Reality monitoring. *Psychol Rev* 1981;**88**:67–85.

Kang M-S, Hong SW, Blake R et al. Visual working memory contaminates perception. *Psychon Bull Rev* 2011;**18**:860–869.

Ko Y, Lau H. A detection theoretic explanation of blindsight suggests a link between conscious perception and metacognition. *Philos Trans R Soc Lond B Biol Sci* 2012;**367**:1401–1411.

Kriete T, Noelle DC, Cohen JD et al. Indirection and symbol-like processing in the prefrontal cortex and basal ganglia. *Proc Natl Acad Sci U S A* 2013;**110**:16390–16395.

Lau H. Consciousness, metacognition, & perceptual reality monitoring. 2019. https://doi.org/10.31234/osf.io/ckbyf.

Lau H, Brown R. The emperor's new phenomenology? The empirical case for conscious experiences without first-order representations. In: A Pautz, D Stoljar (eds), *Blockheads! Essays on Ned Block's philosophy of mind and consciousness.* The MIT Press; 2019; 171–197.

Lau H, Rosenthal D. Empirical support for higher-order theories of conscious awareness. *Trends Cogn Sci* 2011;**15**:365–373.

LeDoux JE, Lau H. Seeing consciousness through the lens of memory. *Curr Biol* 2020;**30**:R1018–R1022.

Mendoza-Halliday D, Martinez-Trujillo JC. Neuronal population coding of perceived and memorized visual features in the lateral prefrontal cortex. *Nat Commun* 2017;**8**:15471.

Muzur A, Pace-Schott EF, Hobson JA. The prefrontal cortex in sleep. *Trends Cogn Sci* 2002;**6**:475–481.

Narayanan NS, Rodnitzky RL, Uc EY. Prefrontal dopamine signaling and cognitive symptoms of Parkinson's disease. *Rev Neurosci* 2013;**24**. https://doi.org/10.1515/revneuro-2013-0004.

Nikolajsen L, Ilkjaer S, Krøner K et al. The influence of preamputation pain on postamputation stump and phantom pain. *Pain* 1997;**72**:393–405.

Onofrj M, Taylor JP, Monaco D et al. Visual hallucinations in PD and Lewy body dementias: Old and new hypotheses. *Behav Neurol* 2013;**27**:479–493.

Oosterhof NN, Tipper SP, Downing PE. Visuo-motor imagery of specific manual actions: A multi-variate pattern analysis fMRI study. *Neuroimage* 2012;**63**:262–271.

Pitcher G. *Theory of Perception*. Princeton University Press, 1971.

Pu Y, Gan Z, Henao R et al. Variational autoencoder for deep learning of images, labels and captions. In Proceedings of the 30th International Conference on Neural Information Processing Systems (NIPS'16). Curran Associates Inc., Red Hook, NY, USA, 2360–2368.

Raichle ME. Neuroscience. The brain's dark energy. *Science* 2006;**314**:1249–1250.

Rasmus A, Valpola H, Honkala M et al. Semi-supervised learning with Ladder networks. In Proceedings of the 28th International Conference on Neural Information Processing Systems - Volume 2 (NIPS'15). MIT Press, Cambridge, MA, USA, 3546–3554.

Richter FR, Cooper RA, Bays PM et al. Distinct neural mechanisms underlie the success, precision, and vividness of episodic memory. *Elife* 2016;**5**. https://doi.org/10.7554/eLife.18260.

Rosenthal D. *Consciousness and Mind*. Oxford University Press, 2005.

Salahub CM, Emrich SM. Tuning perception: Visual working memory biases the quality of visual awareness. *Psychon Bull Rev* 2016;**23**:1854–1859.

Sato W, Kochiyama T, Yoshikawa S et al. Enhanced neural activity in response to dynamic facial expressions of emotion: an fMRI study. *Brain Res Cogn Brain Res* 2004;**20**:81–91.

Sauret W, Lycan WG. Attention and internal monitoring: A farewell to HOP. *Analysis* 2014;**74**:363–370.

Schaeffer DJ, Hori Y, Gilbert KM et al. Divergence of rodent and primate medial frontal cortex functional connectivity. *Proc Natl Acad Sci U S A* 2020;**117**:21681–21689.

Schölvinck ML, Howarth C, Attwell D. The cortical energy needed for conscious perception. *Neuroimage* 2008;**40**:1460–1468.

Segal SJ, Gordon PE. The perky effect revisited: blocking of visual signals by imagery. *Percept Mot Skills* 1969;**28**:791–797.

Segal SJ, Nathan S. The perky effect: Incorporation of an external stimulus into an imagery experience under placebo and control conditions. *Percept Mot Skills* 1964;**18**:385–395.

Siclari F, Baird B, Perogamvros L et al. The neural correlates of dreaming. *Nat Neurosci* 2017;**20**:872–878.

Simons JS, Garrison JR, Johnson MK. Brain mechanisms of reality monitoring. *Trends Cogn Sci* 2017;**21**:462–473.

Singer T, Seymour B, O'Doherty J et al. Empathy for pain involves the affective but not sensory components of pain. *Science* 2004;**303**:1157–1162.

Stolyarova A, Rakhshan M, Hart EE et al. Contributions of anterior cingulate cortex and basolateral amygdala to decision confidence and learning under uncertainty. *Nat Commun* 2019;**10**:4704.

Stumbrys T, Erlacher D, Schredl M. Testing the involvement of the prefrontal cortex in lucid dreaming: A tDCS study. *Conscious Cogn* 2013;**22**:1214–1222.

Taube W, Mouthon M, Leukel C et al. Brain activity during observation and motor imagery of different balance tasks: An fMRI study. *Cortex* 2015;**64**:102–114.

Teng C, Kravitz DJ. Visual working memory directly alters perception. *Nat Hum Behav* 2019;**3**:827–836.

Voss U, Holzmann R, Hobson A et al. Induction of self-awareness in dreams through frontal low current stimulation of gamma activity. *Nat Neurosci* 2014;**17**:810–812.

Zabicki A, de Haas B, Zentgraf K et al. Imagined and executed actions in the human motor system: Testing neural similarity between execution and imagery of actions with a multivariate approach. *Cereb Cortex* 2017;**27**:4523–4536.

Zeman A, Dewar M, Della Sala S. Lives without imagery—Congenital aphantasia. *Cortex* 2015;**73**:378–380.

Zmigrod L, Garrison JR, Carr J et al. The neural mechanisms of hallucinations: A quantitative meta-analysis of neuroimaging studies. *Neurosci Biobehav Rev* 2016;**69**:113–123.

8
Making Ourselves Useful

8.1 Beliefs & Reality

The theory of perceptual reality monitoring (PRM), introduced in Chapter 7, connects two important notions of consciousness: subjective experience, and our rational grasp of reality. The former is what we have focused on so far. But the latter is no less relevant. Studies in the social sciences, psychiatry, and clinical psychology have focused on this notion of consciousness for over a century. To many, that's where the concept of consciousness really comes from, or at least that's what makes the topic so interesting. A theory of consciousness would do well to allow something meaningful to be said about this connection between the two notions.

The local theorist may complain that I'm changing the topic. We set out to understand consciousness in order to say something about the Hard Problem. There, subjective experience is what matters. Rationality does not. But I'm not saying that consciousness is rationality. PRM is about subjective experience, as promised. Nor am I saying that consciousness is what you believe. Rather, it is the mechanism by which you *potentially* form beliefs about what you perceive. These beliefs are rational in the sense that they *feel* justified; it seems to make sense to believe them and to act according to them, at least from the subject's point of view. This is how consciousness is connected to rationality.

The goal of this chapter is to flesh out this connection in more detail. A better understanding of this connection can inform clinical and social applications. It also makes clear why PRM is a "centrist" theory (Chapter 6), that is, a happy medium between extreme options. It accounts for subjective experience, without writing off broader issues like the role of consciousness in cognition and rational behavior. I will also argue that it is only with this more extended version of PRM that we can fully account for the experiences of emotions and volition.

There is an alternative to this line of thinking, which is to say: consciousness is just subjective experience. For those who use the word to refer to anything related to rationality, they are just using the word *entirely* differently. It is true that some words refer to totally different things (e.g., *palm* can refer to

In Consciousness We Trust. Hakwan Lau, Oxford University Press. © Hakwan Lau 2022.
DOI: 10.1093/oso/9780198856771.003.0009

a kind of tree or a part of our hand). But are the notions of "consciousness" in these different contexts really entirely unrelated in such a way? At times many contemporary neuroscientists working on consciousness come close to taking this extreme view. But remember from Chapter 1 Section 1.5, that definitions are never hard and fast matters. There is a cost to defining ourselves into a corner, making ourselves irrelevant to our academic neighbors. As we will see, there is just no need to do so.

8.2 Symbolic Causal Narratives

Rational agents act according to their beliefs and desires. For example, if we desire an apple, and we believe that there is an apple in front of us, we may proceed to grab the apple. But other beliefs are also relevant: For example, is it polite given the social context? How much money would it cost? Could the apples be poisonous?

Some of the relevant beliefs are not perceptual beliefs. They don't concern what we see or otherwise feel at the moment. They may even concern things that do not exist in the concrete, such as social etiquette, money, and the fear of death by poison. And yet they no doubt impact our rational actions and decisions.

Nor are these more abstract beliefs entirely unrelated to our perceptual beliefs. The two sets of beliefs have to somehow hang together in a *coherent way*. If we believe that it is socially inappropriate for someone to grab the apple in the present context, but we see another person doing it, either we doubt the social norm we believe in, or we doubt what we're seeing correctly—or we form the judgment that the person grabbing the apple must be rude. Somehow, we form an overall *story* that is more or less coherent. Things we believe in have to make sense together. They have to roughly "add up."

We can call this coherent web of beliefs our *narrative* of reality. In narratives, things are expressed in causal terms. When we say that President Obama got fired up in a rally and started leading the crowd to cheer, we mean that his enthusiasm *caused* him to act that way, and his action *caused* the crowd to follow. To believe that something is socially inappropriate is to believe that *if* certain norms are violated, there will *then* be certain undesirable consequences. To believe that something is poisonous is to believe that consuming it will *cause* sickness or death.

But causal models are notoriously difficult to build from observations alone. Just because X precedes Y doesn't mean that X causes Y at all; they could be both caused by something else, with the effect on Y just being more delayed.

Or they could be mere coincidences. It would help if we could manipulate X at will. And our actions do impact our world. But as far as the beliefs we just talked about are concerned, we can't move President Obama's level of enthusiasm up and down in order to assess the consequences accordingly. We can't turn a social norm on and off at will to see if people's behavior changes. Sometimes these are stories just told to us. They might have already happened, and there's no room for intervention.

My former colleague at UCLA Judea Pearl has spelled out the logic for building these kinds of models for causal inferences (Pearl and Mackenzie 2018). These models are crucial for counterfactual reasoning. That is an extremely important ingredient for intelligence. To make good decisions, we need more than a grasp of the known facts. We need to be able to think about hypothetical scenarios: For example, *what happens if I try this new solution? What happens if we try something else instead?*

The computational methods proposed by Pearl are elegant, but they also highlight how demanding they are, in terms of the amount of data needed, *if* we are to build the models from the ground up. So, instead, many assumptions need to be made. The role of data is primarily to arbitrate between plausible alternatives. These alternatives can be expressed schematically in some "graphs" (Figure 8.1).

This means that to empirically inform causal reasoning, we probably need to conceptualize the relevant events at a *symbolic* level. Our sensory representations are analog and detailed. For the narrative models to work, we would do well to include only the key facts, and exclude uncertain, noisy information. Some abstraction and simplification are probably needed to summarize things for causal reasoning.

Importantly, the sensory representations driven by imagination and perception may be similar. But at the causal reasoning level they make a world

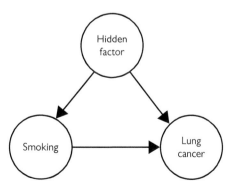

Figure 8.1 An example "graph" representation of what may cause lung cancer

of difference. Some hard and fast decisions need to be made about what the sensory activity really represents before the information is passed on to the narrative level.

This may be how the perceptual reality monitor described in Chapter 7 contributes to our narratives of reality, by boiling down rich perceptual information into something worth believing and thinking about further. In this sense, consciousness may be the "gating" mechanism through which perception impinges on higher cognition.

8.3 Split-Brain Patients & Confabulations

I have not given proof that this is exactly how we represent reality in the brain. In Section 8.2 we went through some engineering considerations as to what may be a plausible general architecture, based on our current knowledge in the computer and cognitive sciences. Ideally, we shall investigate the neurocognitive mechanisms more directly in the future. Some existing work is relevant and congruent (reviewed in LeDoux and Lau 2020). But perhaps just as telling are some classic patient studies.

In split-brain patients with their corpus callosum severed, information could be selectively presented to just one of the hemispheres. When information is presented to the right hemisphere, patients tend not to report being aware of it, because language functions mostly reside on the left hemisphere. However, such information can evidently have an impact on behavior. In one famous study, the patient was asked to pick a picture that was most relevant to what was shown (Volz and Gazzaniga 2017). A snow scene was shown to the (nonconscious) right hemisphere, and a chicken claw was shown to the left hemisphere. The patient picked a shovel. That made sense given the snow scene. But because the patient was not aware of seeing the snow scene, he reported that the shovel was relevant to the chicken claw, because it could be used to clean up the chicken excrements!

This kind of confabulation behavior has been found in other patients too, such as those who suffered from hemispatial neglect. In one study a patient was presented with two houses, the left of which was on fire in one (Marshall and Halligan 1988). Because of the neurological condition, the patient reported that both houses looked similar. However, when asked which house the patient would prefer to live in, the house on fire was avoided. And yet, the patient could not really give a convincing answer to justify the choice.

One interpretation is that the coherence-seeking narrative system can only take into account what one is conscious of (Liu and Lau 2021). When nonconscious information impacts behavior, it creates a difficult situation for the system to make sense of the situation. Hence the confabulatory justifications are somewhat funny. In this sense, our narrative system is often not fully rational, just *quasi*-rational.

I cannot say that these examples provide decisive evidence for a narrative system exactly as described in Section 8.2. But my point here is more modest: something akin to a coherence-seeking narrative system probably exists in some form. To fully understand consciousness, we would do well to learn more about how such a system may interact with subjective experiences.

8.4 Narratives as "Consciousness"

Why should we care about these narratives? One reason is that there is a long tradition in the social and mental health sciences of identifying this narrative mechanism as "consciousness" itself.

When Marxist theorists talk about "false consciousness," it is not about sensory hallucinations (Lukacs 1972). It is about how certain people fail to comprehend reality correctly, and to act rationally according to how resources and power are actually allocated. They may see the same physical objects and hear the same sounds as the ruling class. They see the same movement of goods, food, and money. But they misunderstand the underlying causes and effects. They underestimate the far-reaching consequences *if* they were to collectively stop working for the ruling class. Their consciousness is "false" because they got the causal narratives wrong.

Likewise, when the great sociologist Émile Durkheim wrote about "collective consciousness," it referred to the common narratives of reality shared between members of a group (2014). It was not about the science fiction-like possibility that different people may merge together into a single conscious entity, as if they could share a singular stream of subjective experiences.

Importantly, according to these views our narratives are functionally relevant. They impact our rational decision-making. Getting the narratives wrong is detrimental to our bargaining behavior. It causes us to be exploited. It can make social cooperation difficult.

In the psychiatry and clinical psychology tradition, "consciousness" is also often understood in terms of these narratives. In particular, psychoanalysts claim that there is an "unconscious" mind that is opaque to direct cognitive access and control (Alexander 1948). But the "conscious" mind is not equated with only ongoing sensory experiences either. Whatever one can access through direct introspection, including abstract knowledge, are considered "conscious." So, like the political theorists, they also often use the term *con-sciousness* to refer to our rational (or rationalized) narratives. But psychoana-lysts suggest that the "unconscious" mind is just as capable of sophisticated forms of reasoning, as if it also has its own independent narrative system of some sort.

Nevertheless, psychoanalysis has not become an empirically successful sci-ence. This leaves us doubting if there really are such things as fully fledged "nonconscious" narrative mechanisms. The view I propose is that there isn't.

However, on a more practical level, these two questions are also left open: *are there "nonconscious" ways to change our "conscious" narratives?* And how about the opposite: *can our "conscious" narratives impact "nonconscious" processes too?* Below I will argue positively for both: our "conscious" narratives and at least some "nonconscious" processes influence each other. This is true especially for affective processes, which often seem to happen outside of our conscious control. This may in a sense suggest that the psychoanalysts aren't entirely wrong. Not only does this matter for our theory of consciousness, but also these questions have clinical and societal implications too.

Because of this tricky terminological issue of the different usages in dif-ferent fields, I will put "conscious" and "nonconscious" in quotations, as I did above, when I refer to this notion of (quasi-)rational narratives that guide de-liberate actions, rather than subjective experiences (our default usage of the term *consciousness*).

8.5 Self, Actions, & Responsibility

One of the most common and stubborn misunderstandings against PRM, and its higher-order relatives, is that we overintellectualize consciousness. The charge is that we conflate simple subjective experiences with explicit intro-spection about oneself (Malach 2011). But the criticism is misplaced because the theory does not actually assume anything like that (Lau and Rosenthal 2011). The self-monitoring mechanism hypothesized in Chapter 7 is auto-matic and implicit (Sections 7.8 and 7.9). That is, some mechanism in your prefrontal cortex needs to know the dynamics of your sensory activity in order to make a perceptual decision. But you *as a person* do not need to make an effort to do so. Conscious experiences just happen to you, even if you don't try to think about them.

But how, then, do we account for our explicit sense of self-awareness? Certainly, people can introspect and explicitly think about themselves too. The narrative system proposed here can perhaps accommodate this because one of its main functions is to deal with the challenging problem of causal reasoning. We think of ourselves as causal agents. We believe that our actions and decisions have causal consequences. In Chapter 5 we pointed out that empirically this is actually a somewhat open-ended question; our sense of agency may well be partially reconstructed after the facts. Nevertheless, regardless of whether our conscious intentions are causal, we no doubt believe that they are. One plausible view is that this comes from our higher-level narratives about ourselves, rather than directly from the motor control system. Truthfully or otherwise, we model ourselves *as* a causal agent in our self-narrative (Laurie Paul, Tomer Ullman, Julian Freitas, Josh Tenenbaum, personal communication).

This is another reason why understanding this narrative system is so important. Philosophical theories often link our sense of free will and moral responsibility to consciousness. But it is unclear if subjective experience per se is the relevant notion (Levy 2014). Instead, our overall sense of agency may arise at the narrative level. This may be why it is relatively malleable (Chapter 5 Section 5.3). And yet, it does not mean that our sense of agency is necessarily always constructed after the facts, as a mere illusion. That is because the narrative system can have causal impacts on both our subjective experiences and rational behavior. As such, disturbances in this sense of agency can have devastating effects, as, for example, observed in psychosis.

8.6 Schizophrenia the Really Hard Problem

Schizophrenia is a severe mental illness that affects as many as close to 1% of the global population (Saha et al. 2005; Schultz, North, and Shields 2007). Many people think of it as *the* disorder of consciousness, probably because of the symptoms of psychosis. We already addressed the possible mechanisms for sensory hallucination in Sections 7.8 and 7.9. But psychosis can also involve the loss of sense of agency, as well as various forms of delusions at a higher-cognitive level. Why do these symptoms often occur together in the same patients?

Chris Frith argued that one underlying mechanism for psychosis may be that patients fail to accurately anticipate the consequences of their self-generated (mental) actions (1992). Accordingly, the sensory consequences become unexpectedly salient and, therefore, sometimes are mistakenly attributed to being caused by external forces. This elegantly accounts for the variety of symptoms, from hallucinations to loss of agency, and the delusory belief that thoughts have been "inserted" into one's minds. In all cases, the idea is that the patients themselves actually generated the imagery, action, or thought. But their brains failed to recognize that fact.

Our account here is similar. But here we factor the symptoms into two levels: the sensory and the cognitive (narrative). As we have discussed in Sections 7.8 and 7.9, these two levels may depend on partially overlapping mechanisms in the prefrontal cortex. Hallucinations, which are mostly auditory in schizophrenia, have early sensory correlates. But they are probably also caused, at least in part, by failures of the perceptual reality monitor. The "discriminator," as described in Chapter 7, mistakes noise or inner speech for external voices. This accounts for the symptoms at the sensory level.

At the narrative level of higher-cognitive reasoning, I suspect a wider variety of more complex problems may arise in psychosis. As mentioned in Section 8.2, the role of the reality monitors may be to select and simplify information for causal reasoning. When they fail to provide reliable information for this computationally demanding process, different sorts of catastrophic errors can occur. In terms of signal processing, we can say that for causal narrative reasoning, noise is *multiplicative* rather than additive. That is to say, on this analytic and symbolic level, we can't always average out the noise like we do in early sensory processing. Overall, a certain degree of coherence may still be maintained, even when the inputs are noisy, leading to confabulatory responses. But the errors on this level may become so unpredictable and bizarre that, ultimately, they may impact one's general ability to think and behave rationally.

This way, we can more easily explain why hallucinations do not always co-occur with psychosis. But one problem is that this account is much less parsimonious than Frith's elegant model. But indeed, the point here is exactly that more effort in understanding the narrative mechanism is needed. Fortunately, there is a relatively familiar way for us to intuitively appreciate and perhaps even manipulate the operations at this causal narrative level: through our language and culture.

The medical anthropologist Tanya Luhrmann has described that, in different cultures, certain individuals apparently experience auditory "hallucinations," even though they are never formally diagnosed as such (Luhrmann et al. 2015). Instead, many of them relish in their ability to "hear voices," which they consider an important part of their societal role and religious practice. In many cases, this difference in cultural beliefs allows these individuals to enjoy productive and rewarding lives without the stigma of "madness."

Perhaps these reports suggest that the sensory and cognitive components of schizophrenia are indeed somewhat independent; for these individuals, the "hallucinations" do not simply go away, even though the problems are somewhat resolved at the "narrative" level. Arguably, one could say that these individuals still suffer from undiagnosed "delusions." But this runs the risk of unfairly imposing our own views on otherwise well-functioning people, who do not consider themselves to be suffering.

Can these thought-provoking findings translate into treatments in the clinic? Unfortunately, the effectiveness of current psychotherapy for psychosis is somewhat limited. Antipsychotic drugs targeting prefrontal dopaminergic functions remain the standard prescription. For interventions at the psychological or narrative level, there have been some exciting recent developments (Craig et al. 2018), but we await to see robust effects replicated in large-scale studies. It is also possible that our narratives are so embedded within our culture that changing them would take more than the patient's brief interaction with a therapist—at least for the moment, until we can understand the narrative mechanisms better.

Meanwhile, there may be another venue where psychology may help. If our view is right, even if there is some degree of independence between the sensory and cognitive levels, the former may be more primary; subjective experiences are associated with the gating mechanisms for downstream narrative processing. As such, disturbances at the narrative level are perhaps typically caused by faulty inputs from the sensory level. Because the reality monitoring and perceptual metacognitive mechanisms are relatively better understood, one can develop simple psychophysical tasks to test for their functioning in both health and disease (Hoven et al. 2019). Along these lines, for example, Koller and Cannon (2021) have recently found that paranoid individuals indeed showed specific deficits in metacognitive processing in recognition memory tasks. Given present knowledge, we do not expect to be able to fix these mechanisms with precision whenever they break down. But patients with schizophrenia often first go through what is called a "prodromal" stage, before the symptoms become fully fledged (Larson, Walker, and Compton 2010). Early detection with such psychophysical tasks can facilitate preventive treatment.

8.7 How Affective Experiences & Narratives Interact

The above discussion suggests that social stigma may be one reason why psychotherapy alone may not resolve all the conflicts at the narrative level. In modern societies, unfortunately, people often react to psychotic behavior with strong negative emotions, such as distress or fear. This is so despite the fact that, in the absence of substance abuse problems, psychosis alone isn't strongly associated with violent behavior (Fazel et al. 2009). Given this cultural bias, it may be difficult from the patient's point of view to see things as going alright.

Specifically, this breaks down into three key points: i) emotions influence narrative processing; ii) narratives influence emotions; and iii) emotions can be contagious. That is to say, for a patient suffering from psychosis in modern societies, it may be difficult to form a very positive self-narrative because one usually goes through significant emotional distress. Some of this negative affect may come from other people, who do not see the situation in a very positive light. But all the same, the resulting emotion may also influence the patient's own feelings toward their condition. Let us unpack these points.

The first point may be straightforward. The narratives we've been discussing are often self-narratives. When we feel afraid, typically the only immediate belief that we can form is just that we are afraid; we may not know why or what really causes our fear. The causal analysis may take place at least in part at the narrative level. In seeking coherence, we tend not to accept easily that we are frightened for no reason. Instead, the mind seeks plausible explanations.

The social psychologist Jonathan Haidt has given the analogy that our "conscious" decision-making is a bit like riding an elephant (2012). As "rational" agents, we'd like to think we are in control of our emotions. But the slow and powerful animal we are riding has its own mind. We can nudge it toward our desired directions here and there. But in the end, we are often just going along for the ride. We make up post hoc rationalizations to justify our "decisions." But maybe emotions are really the driving forces.

This idea traces back to David Hume, and has a huge influence on the social sciences, maybe in particular in political theory (Gauthier 1979). Its wisdom rings just as true today: much of our political and moral debates do come down to affect, often more than we realize. If people feel a certain way about certain political issues, they may contrive to come up with the arguments to support how they feel. This probably happens more often than we are prepared to admit. In this sense, the logical arguments are secondary, and it is emotion that is truly fundamental to, for example, social change or elections.

But as Pizarro and Bloom (2003) have pointed out, the influence can go the other way too. Narratives at the cognitive level can also influence emotions (i.e., narratives influence emotions, the second point above). Our emotional reactions to the same set of sensory events often depend on how we see the overall narrative. If someone says something rude and aggressive to us, our reactions can be anything from anger, fear, guilt, or remorse, to disinterested sadness. It all depends on how we interpret the situation, the history of what happened, and what we expect may happen next. It may involve counterfactual reasoning too, e.g., *What if I tell the person to calm down? How likely would it work? Or how about I just run?* Our preliminary answers to questions like these seem to determine how we feel. If such implicit thinking does take place, however imperfect it may be, it must happen pretty fast.

That is to say, emotions are not just simple "gut reactions"; we should not confuse simple physiological reactions with full-blown emotions. When we are physiologically aroused, we are sometimes just as likely to be scared or falling in love. To find out which is the case, our cognitive understanding of the context matters (Schachter and Singer 1962).

Finally, it is well-known that emotions are contagious (Hatfield, Cacioppo, and Rapson 1993; the third point above). Some may think this reflects mostly automatic mimicry. When people look afraid, we may sometimes feel scared too, without thinking. But perhaps there is also some rationale to contagion, even at the narrative level. Let's say you visit a new country and you find that people are generally mortified by the sight of squirrels. Instead, they seem to find rats cute. Perhaps it makes sense for you to draw the inference: maybe squirrels are poisonous there, and rats are relatively hygienic and harmless? Maybe eventually you will—and should—learn to be afraid of those (hypothetically) deadly squirrels too.

Despite the "quasi-rational" nature of these ways of interactions, the logic isn't always so transparent to us. Therefore, we may overestimate how "conscious" our narrative system really is. Our narratives are often influenced by emotions in ways rather opaque to us, beyond our control. Although we have the ability to regulate our emotions at will to some extent, its reach is not unlimited (Gross 2002).

8.8 Affective Learning, Homophily, & Culture

The limits of our emotional insights and regulation may be related to one of BF Skinner's arguments for behaviorism. Late in his career, Skinner speculated about "consciousness," and even openly explored Freudian ideas (Overskeid 2007). But prior to that, in a debate against the role of conscious thoughts in psychology, he mentioned that the behaviorist's point was not that these high-level constructs are unobservable and, therefore, cannot be studied (Blanshard and Skinner 1967). Rather, the worry was that they may not provide as much leverage for systematically predicting and controlling behavior.

In contrast, since Pavlov, psychology has made tremendous progress on our understanding of the mechanisms underlying the learning of simple emotions like fear (Rescorla 1988). In general, these mechanisms follow the principles of associative conditioning. When a neutral stimulus is consistently paired with something frightening, we learn to be afraid of the neutral stimulus too.

Of particular interest is one form of conditioning called vicarious learning (Olsson, Knapska, and Lindström 2020), which we have already described in our squirrel and rats example in Section 8.7. The idea is that we may learn to react with certain emotions by observing how others react to the same stimuli or situations.

Because of the ways narratives and emotions interact, through vicarious learning, different people can learn to synchronize their narratives too. This is somewhat turning the problem on its head. But I suspect it is actually a rather common phenomenon. For example, when I was only 9 years old, I saw the news on TV about a peaceful protest being cracked down on by an authoritarian regime, leading to a massacre. No doubt that back then, I had not thought through the concepts of justice, liberty, power, and mercy. But I distinctly remember learning then that anger and sadness were the "appropriate" social reactions. If someone reacted to the same tragic news with elation and joy, or sheer indifference, that person would no doubt be shunned by the people I love and respect. Without a word spoken, this already helped strangers ensure that they share a similar narrative of what really happened.

Of course, in society, we can talk through our narratives too. We can debate about them, and make sure we're all on the same page. But the full narratives are often complex, and our communication skills may be limited. On the other hand, the vicarious learning of emotions is based on simple and robust mechanisms (Olsson, Knapska, and Lindström 2020). Additionally, there is the factor of homophily. That is, we tend to sort ourselves into groups of similar people. We hang out with people we find agreeable. As I just mentioned in the example in the last paragraph, our emotional responses probably play a significant role in helping us identify like-minded people too.

These may be some of the ways through which our cognitive processes are so powerfully modulated by culture (Heyes 1993). Because of the mechanisms of associative learning, the very simple acts of sharing a meal or watching a movie together may have more impact on our "consciousness" than we may intuitively expect. Linguistic communication is no doubt important. But shared subjective experiences also contribute greatly to how common narratives are formed.

8.9 "Consciousness" Fast Versus Slow?

So, we have gone through some key concepts, regarding how "consciousness" (narratives) and consciousness (subjective affective experience) may interact. It may be useful to think of how this relates to similar models too.

For example, the Nobel laureate Daniel Kahneman distinguished between a fast (System 1) and a slow (System 2) thinking system (2011). The former is relatively intuitive, automatic, and emotion-like. The latter is more rational and analytical. The narrative system we've discussed so far may map well to Kahneman's System 2.

Likewise, in the literature on the computational models of learning, there is also a distinction between model-free and model-based learning (Dayan and Berridge 2014). In model-free learning, the causal relations between events aren't explicitly represented. The learning is more akin to statistical associations, driven by the principles Pavlovian (and Skinnerian) conditioning described in Section 8.8. Model-based learning is more similar to the narrative system described so far.

One caveat is that these views are typically not so strongly committed to the nature of subjective experience. Subjective experience may or may not accompany System 1 (i.e., fast, intuitive) reasoning; nonconscious representations (in the sense of lacking subjective experience) and unreflected conscious percepts are both likely governed by the same simple model-free associative learning principles. But if a perceptual event is nonconscious, according to PRM it will probably not be selected (by the perceptual reality monitor) for making downstream impact on System 2 or complex, model-based learning.

Another difference between these views and PRM is that some may see Systems 1 and 2 as working in parallel. Likewise, model-based and model-free learning systems may also operate side-by-side, in some form of competition or cooperation. On PRM though, the narrative system is a late-stage process downstream in a hierarchical architecture, relative to early perceptual processes. That is, it takes selected early perceptual information as input. However, this late-stage process probably also feeds back to early sensory processing (LeDoux and Lau 2020). So, simple perceptual experiences may show some level of coherence too.

We already argued for this kind of feedback modulation in the case of emotions earlier in Section 8.7. In the case of perceptual experiences, one anecdotal consideration is that dreams also tend to be somewhat structured; the subjective experiences in dreams do not seem like random sensory "noises." One explanation could be that the coherence comes from the narrative system.

If that's true even during sleep, perhaps subjective experiences can never be completely understood in isolation from the narrative mechanisms too.

The last point may be one reason why we should reject behaviorism, despite Skinner's argument described in the Section 8.8. To change psychological behavior, it may be useful to target the associative learning mechanisms for affective responses, which are better understood. However, there are occasions where the narratives themselves play important causal roles too, or they may be the very targets we want to ultimately change. In Sections 8.10-8.12, we will quickly review some examples as to how we can apply these concepts in clinical and societal contexts.

8.10 Fear & Trauma

Let us start with cases in which it is desirable to reduce the intensity of some emotional experiences. People who went through life-threatening traumas may experience "flashbacks" of the incidents, which can trigger very unpleasant and intense experiences of fear. Sometimes, it is as if the trauma is being "relived." But these are not the only possible symptoms. Posttraumatic stress disorder (PTSD) can also impact a person's cognition, including one's self-image and autobiographical memories (Sutherland and Bryant 2008). In severe cases, it can lead to suicidal thoughts and behavior. As such, psychotherapy focusing on the cognitive or narrative levels is evidently helpful in some cases (Kar 2011).

That said, a common treatment is (some variant of) exposure therapy, which we discussed briefly in Sections 5.12 and 5.13. The idea comes from simple Pavlovian conditioning principles. If a trauma-related cue (e.g., a specific weapon) is presented repeatedly without harm, one may "unlearn" previously associated fear with the cue. Essentially, the focus is on prenarrative-level sensory processing. In Sections 5.12 and 5.13, we specifically described a way to achieve this nonconsciously, using the method of decoded neurofeedback (DecNef).

Why may this kind of treatment be effective? Theoretically, it has been suggested that the traumatic events may be encoded into two kinds of memory representations: sensory and conceptual (Brewin, Dalgleish, and Joseph 1996). In PTSD the sensory representations may dominate, which accounts for the relatively uncontrolled nature of the memory process. When the memories are involuntarily "recalled," they seem intrusive and "relived" as if they are presently occurring. They seem to be disconnected with narrative-level contextual processing. Or they may be so dominant they "hijack" normal cognitive processing. If that is correct, it may be advantageous to selectively target the abnormally dominant early sensory associative mechanisms.

In this theoretical context, there are predictions we can test too. If conscious and nonconscious processes operate entirely in parallel, targeting nonconscious sensory mechanisms may never change the conscious subjective experiences (Taschereau-Dumouchel, Liu, and Lau 2018). As we mentioned in Section 5.13, indeed currently we do not yet know if methods such as DecNef can affect more than physiological responses. However, if conscious and nonconscious mechanisms are common at the early sensory level, we may expect DecNef to eventually be able to change subjective experience too. From there, perhaps even narrative-level processing could be impacted. So, this is an empirically open-ended question that we may be able to address in the near future.

8.11 Placebo Pain & the "Crisis of Neurology"

Contrast PTSD with chronic pain. The latter may seem a lot less "psychological." But pain is also subject to placebo manipulations (Price, Finniss, and Benedetti 2008). That is, the sheer idea that they are being treated can paradoxically reduce pain, even in the absence of a real treatment. This effect is in fact very robust and common, which is why modern medicine generally adopts double-blinded procedures; in establishing the effectiveness of a new treatment, we need to rule out these powerful placebo effects. Using neuroimaging, it has been shown that the placebo effect of pain relief was correlated with reduced activity in early somatosensory regions too (Atlas and Wager 2012). So, narrative-level cognitive processes seem to influence pain experience.

The blurriness of the boundary between the psychological and early sensorimotor processing is highlighted in another class of disorders that are sometimes labeled by neurologists as "functional" or "psychogenic" (Edwards, Stone, and Lang 2014). For example, in functional movement disorders a patient may make unwanted and apparently involuntary tics. However, anatomically there are no identifiable causes. Standard physiological measures like the electroencephalogram may also detect no problems. Intriguingly, in some cases when the patients are distracted, the tics may go away. This seems to suggest that the issue is "psychiatric" or "psychological." But, in fact, these patients are typically perfectly lucid and seem to have no trouble making rational decisions.

There has been some evidence that functional movement disorders are linked to early childhood trauma (Kranick et al. 2011). But certainly most cases of traumatic experiences do not lead to such selective and unique impact on the motor system. The mechanisms are currently unclear. And yet functional movement disorders are extremely common, affecting up to 30% of all patients seeking help for movement disorders (Hallett 2019). Our limited perspective on this widespread clinical phenomenon has led some authors to describe this as a "crisis of neurology." There's an urgent need to better understand how high-level psychological and cognitive factors influence basic neurological symptoms.

8.12 Economics & Political Polarization

Earlier, in Section 8.7, I mentioned the ideas of Haidt and Hume, according to which much of our moral and political reasoning may be driven by intuitions and emotions. But I also pointed out that narratives may also influence our emotions.

In some ways, in politics, often it is the narrative that ultimately matters. My former colleague at UCLA Davide Panagia calls it *narratocracy* (2009); in a sense, society is governed by the stories we share. Take racism as an example. Some people may have a gut feeling that it is dangerous to be in a neighborhood populated by people of a different race. Statistically, perhaps this is actually true in some cases. The rate of violent crime may be higher there. In this sense, our "nonconscious" associative learning mechanisms might have picked up nothing but factual information. But the important questions to ask are: What causes the higher crime rate in the first place? Have those people of the said different race been given the same opportunities? Have they been treated fairly? These questions involve causal reasoning and can perhaps only be resolved at the narrative level.

The Nobel Prize–winning economist Robert Shiller (2017) also recognizes the power of narratives in driving economic events. He likened many major changes in the financial market to pandemics. Narratives can indeed go viral, leading to mass fear or optimism, which, ultimately, can have major impacts on the stock market and beyond. Interestingly, they also fade away in time, as would be predicted by epidemiological models.

But of course, figuring out these narratives are at times messy; especially because we cannot do experiments on historical events. In the end, we may just sort ourselves into our very own echo chambers of choice, which gives us a sense of belonging but are none closer to the truth. Another former colleague at UCLA Jared Diamond (2019) has opined that the breakdown of face-to-face communication may be one factor in why modern politics is so polarized, especially in the United States. Different groups simply no longer see the same reality; their narratives are no longer in sync.

As I suggested earlier (Section 8.8), the simple act of sharing a meal or watching a movie together may well help us sync up our "consciousness" in ways we don't intuitively expect. Nevertheless ... if only things were this simple. Our current understanding of this putative narrative system is limited. How narratives can affect society, and how they interact with consciousness, remain active areas of research within the social sciences (Clough and Halley 2007; Clough 2008; Hoggett and Thompson 2012). Recent work on using a cognitive neuroscience approach to understand the relationship between metacognition and political polarization seems especially promising (Rollwage et al. 2019).

8.13 Chapter Ending Remarks: Freud, Marx, and Panpsychic Qualia

This chapter covered a lot of ground, but, admittedly, I was only able to do it superficially. It may seem like I'm going against the very premise of this book, which is to argue for an empirically grounded account of consciousness. Much of what is said in this chapter is speculative.

But the purpose here is exactly to bring out this fact: so much is at stake, and yet we know so little.

Historically, the notion of "consciousness"—as in the sense of our rational grasp of reality—has not received a lack of attention. Rather, many great scholars have written insightfully on the topic. Unfortunately, Marxist ideas stimulated real-world "experiments" that did not turn out well; the so-called communist revolutions have led to atrocities still felt today. In the case of the Freudians, it is unclear if empirical truthfulness was ever a priority (Eysenck 1991; Crews 2017).

One important lesson, though, is that Freud's writing remains just as eloquent and stimulating today, and continues to impact the arts and humanities, as well as popular culture. All the same, the sheer lack of empirical rigor alone has attracted tremendous backlash, stifling mental health research for decades (Eysenck 1991). Great ideas can sometimes cause great harm.

Accordingly, many rigorous scientists choose to avoid the topic altogether. It may be correct to point out that one ought not to throw the baby out with the bathwater. But guilt by association is a common phenomenon.

In the introduction, we discussed the "revival" in the 1990s. But is our "new" science of consciousness speaking to these historically important issues in the social and clinical sciences? Are we restoring the balance or merely shifting the attention further away?

Meanwhile, "consciousness" continues to be discussed, with or without our empirical input. In clinical assessment of mental illnesses, self-reports are often treated as supplementary information, giving way to more "rigorous" and "objective" biomarker approaches (forthcoming review w/ Ledoux et al). But these biomarkers are not always in concordance with self-reported subjective experiences (Taschereau-Dumouchel, Kawato, and Lau 2020). And yet, one of our primary goals should be to make the subjects *feel* better. Besides reducing excessive physiological responses, we also want their pain and fear to go away *subjectively*. Our lack of meaningful engagement in these areas means that ultimately the patients are the ones who suffer.

Ironically, those who favor scientifically untestable notions of "pure qualia" over "consciousness" do not really sidestep the issues. By defining consciousness a priori in nonfunctional terms, they cut themselves off from any chance of being able to make meaningful connections to the social and clinical sciences. By not keeping their empirical tallies straight, they also risk making the very same mistakes that ultimately brought down the Freudian empire.

My hope is to convince you that we can avoid this "double fault." The theory of perceptual reality monitoring (PRM) can be related to "consciousness" as we traditionally understand it in other disciplines. Much work still needs to be done. But here I have sketched out how these connections can at least be made and further studied in principle; subjective experience and our (quasi-) rational narratives causally interact with each other, in systematic ways. It may therefore be advantageous to understand both in conjunction, rather than in isolation. This is especially so if we intend to manipulate either people's subjective experiences or their narratives; sometimes it may be most effective to change one by influencing the other, or we may try to target both at the same time for potential synergistic effects. For many basic psychological phenomena, mental disorders, and societal problems, our understanding will ever remain incomplete if we do not also consider the narrative mechanisms.

Given the potential utility of these applications, it would be unwise for us to define our discipline into isolated obscurity. Fans of panpsychism or other forms of nonfunctional "qualia" may challenge that we focus too much on high-level cognition, betraying our "roots." Is PRM capable of answering their philosophical concerns too? We will address this in Chapter 9, our next and final chapter.

References

Alexander F. *Fundamentals of Psychoanalysis*. W.W Norton, 1948.

Atlas LY, Wager TD. How expectations shape pain. *Neurosci Lett* 2012;**520**:140–148.

Blanshard B, Skinner BF. The problem of consciousness: A debate. *Philos Phenomenol Res* 1967;**27**:317–337.

Brewin CR, Dalgleish T, Joseph S. A dual representation theory of posttraumatic stress disorder. *Psychol Rev* 1996;**103**:670–686.

Clough PT. The affective turn: Political economy, biomedia and bodies. *Theory, Culture & Society* 2008;**25**:1–22.

Clough PT, Halley J. *The Affective Turn: Theorizing the Social*. Duke University Press, 2007.

Craig TK, Rus-Calafell M, Ward T et al. AVATAR therapy for auditory verbal hallucinations in people with psychosis: A single-blind, randomised controlled trial. *Lancet Psychiatry* 2018;**5**:31–40.

Crews F. *Freud: The Making of an Illusion*. Profile Books, 2017.

Dayan P, Berridge KC. Model-based and model-free Pavlovian reward learning: Revaluation, revision, and revelation. *Cogn Affect Behav Neurosci* 2014;**14**:473–492.

Diamond J. *Upheaval: Turning Points for Nations in Crisis*. Little Brown, 2019.

Durkheim E. *The Division of Labor in Society*. Simon & Schuster, 2014.

Edwards MJ, Stone J, Lang AE. From psychogenic movement disorder to functional movement disorder: It's time to change the name. *Mov Disord* 2014;**29**:849–852.

Eysenck HJ. *Decline and Fall of the Freudian Empire*. Transaction Publishers, 1991.

Fazel S, Gulati G, Linsell L et al. Schizophrenia and violence: Systematic review and meta-analysis. *PLOS Med* 2009;**6**:e1000120.

Frith CD. *The Cognitive Neuropsychology of Schizophrenia*. Psychology Press, 1992.

Gauthier D. David Hume, contractarian. *Philos Rev* 1979;**88**:3–38.

Gross JJ. Emotion regulation: Affective, cognitive, and social consequences. *Psychophysiology* 2002;**39**:281–291.

Haidt J. *The Righteous Mind: Why Good People Are Divided by Politics and Religion*. Knopf Doubleday Publishing Group, 2012.

Hallett M. Functional movement disorders: Is the crisis resolved? *Mov Disord* 2019;**34**:971–974.

Hatfield E, Cacioppo JT, Rapson RL. Emotional contagion. *Curr Dir Psychol Sci* 1993;**2**:96–100.

Heyes CM. Imitation, culture and cognition. *Anim Behav* 1993;**46**:999–1010.

Hoggett P, Thompson S. *Politics and the Emotions: The Affective Turn in Contemporary Political Studies*. Bloomsbury Publishing, 2012.

Hoven M, Lebreton M, Engelmann JB et al. Abnormalities of confidence in psychiatry: An overview and future perspectives. *Transl Psychiatry* 2019;**9**:268.

Kahneman D. *Thinking, Fast and Slow*. Macmillan, 2011.

Kar N. Cognitive behavioral therapy for the treatment of post-traumatic stress disorder: A review. *Neuropsychiatr Dis Treat* 2011;**7**:167–181.

Koller WN, Cannon TD. Paranoia is associated with impaired novelty detection and overconfidence in recognition memory judgments. *J Abnorm Psychol* 2021. 130;3:273–285 https://doi.org/10.1037/abn0000664.

Kranick S, Ekanayake V, Martinez V et al. Psychopathology and psychogenic movement disorders. *Mov Disord* 2011;**26**:1844–1850.

Larson MK, Walker EF, Compton MT. Early signs, diagnosis and therapeutics of the prodromal phase of schizophrenia and related psychotic disorders. *Expert Rev Neurother* 2010;**10**:1347–1359.

Lau H, Rosenthal D. The higher-order view does not require consciously self-directed introspection: Response to Malach. *Trends Cogn Sci* 2011;**15**:508–509.

LeDoux JE, Lau H. Seeing consciousness through the lens of memory. *Curr Biol* 2020;**30**:R1018–R1022.

Levy N. *Consciousness and Moral Responsibility*. Oxford University Press, 2014.

Liu K, Lau H. A framework for understanding agency. In: PW Kalivas, MP Paulus, JR Lupp (eds), *Intrusive Thinking: From Molecules to Free Will*. Vol 30, pp. 229–245. MIT Press, 2021.

Luhrmann TM, Padmavati R, Tharoor H et al. Hearing voices in different cultures: A social kindling hypothesis. *Top Cogn Sci* 2015;**7**:646–663.

Lukacs G. *History and Class Consciousness: Studies in Marxist Dialectics*. MIT Press, 1972.

Malach R. Conscious perception and the frontal lobes: Comment on Lau and Rosenthal. *Trends Cogn Sci* 2011;**15**:507; author reply 508–509.

Marshall JC, Halligan PW. Blindsight and insight in visuo-spatial neglect. *Nature* 1988;**336**:766–767.

Olsson A, Knapska E, Lindström B. The neural and computational systems of social learning. *Nat Rev Neurosci* 2020;**21**:197–212.

Overskeid G. Looking for Skinner and finding Freud. *Am Psychol* 2007;**62**:590–595.

Panagia D. *The Political Life of Sensation*. Duke University Press, 2009.

Pearl J, Mackenzie D. *The Book of Why: The New Science of Cause and Effect*. Basic Books, 2018.

Pizarro DA, Bloom P. The intelligence of the moral intuitions: comment on Haidt (2001). *Psychol Rev 2003*;**110**:193–196; discussion 197–198.

Price DD, Finniss DG, Benedetti F. A comprehensive review of the placebo effect: Recent advances and current thought. *Annu Rev Psychol* 2008;**59**:565–590.

Rescorla RA. Behavioral studies of Pavlovian conditioning. *Annu Rev Neurosci* 1988;**11**:329–352.

Rollwage M, Zmigrod L, de-Wit L et al. What underlies political polarization? A manifesto for computational political psychology. *Trends Cogn Sci* 2019;**23**:820–822.

Saha S, Chant D, Welham J et al. A systematic review of the prevalence of schizophrenia. *PLOS Med* 2005;**2**:e141.

Schachter S, Singer JE. Cognitive, social, and physiological determinants of emotional state. *Psychol Rev* 1962;**69**:379–399.

Schultz SH, North SW, Shields CG. *Schizophrenia: A Review.* 2007. American family physician. 75(12):1821–1829.

Shiller RJ. Narrative economics. *Am Econ Rev* 2017;**107**:967–1004.

Sutherland K, Bryant RA. Autobiographical memory and the self-memory system in posttraumatic stress disorder. *J Anxiety Disord* 2008;**22**:555–560.

Taschereau-Dumouchel V, Kawato M, Lau H. Multivoxel pattern analysis reveals dissociations between subjective fear and its physiological correlates. *Mol Psychiatry* 2020;**25**:2342–2354.

Taschereau-Dumouchel V, Liu K-Y, Lau H. Unconscious psychological treatments for physiological survival circuits. *Curr Opin Behav Sci* 2018;**24**:62–68.

Vincent Taschereau-Dumouchel, Matthias Michel, Hakwan Lau, Stefan Hofmann, Joseph LeDoux (in press). Putting the 'Mental' Back in 'Mental Disorders': A Perspective from Research on Fear and Anxiety. Molecular Psychiatry.

Volz LJ, Gazzaniga MS. Interaction in isolation: 50 years of insights from split-brain research. *Brain* 2017;**140**:2051–2060.

9

What of the Hard Problem?

9.1 What a Conscious Experience Is Like

Some readers may feel that we have thus far left out the single most important issue: the qualitative aspects of subjective experience.

To many, this Hard Problem—of accounting for the subjective, phenomenological nature of conscious experience—is why we are here in this business in the first place. To some, the supposed deep conceptual mystery is a given. But at times, we also struggle to explain to the uninitiated what the problem really is, without resorting to some philosophical jargon.

It may be telling that one of the most useful phrases in these situations is "what it is like" to have a certain experience (Nagel 1974). We explain to our friends: there is *something it is like* to be in that sharp pain in the finger. That horrible feeling is much more than a piece of information telling you that something is wrong with your finger. It *feels like something* to be in that brain state. Accounting for that "what-it-is-like-ness" in objective scientific terms is the Hard Problem.

9.2 A Structural-Relational View

So what is it like to feel that sharp pain in the finger? Well, it feels somewhat like a dull pain, but is more pinpointed, more concentrated, right? It is not exactly like a dull pain, but it certainly is closer to that than to a gentle stroke. Another way to put it may be to say that the sharp pain at the tip of my index finger is very much like the same pain in my thumb. The locations are different, but the subjective *quality* of the pain is similar. Neither is it like the taste of baked potatoes at all. Nor is the pain anything like the sound of the cello. But if you force me to make an auditory analogy, it is probably somewhat more like the scream of a cat rather than the sound of waves in the ocean.

That is to say, in describing the qualitative character of a conscious experience, the best we can do is often to relate and compare it with other experiences we've had. In fact, perhaps this is not just a matter of communication.

In Consciousness We Trust. Hakwan Lau, Oxford University Press. © Hakwan Lau 2022.
DOI: 10.1093/oso/9780198856771.003.0010

When we think about what an experience is like, we can't help but think in these terms too. As soon as we imagine what the experience is like, comparing it with other experiences seems intuitive. Even when we don't explicitly make these comparisons, perhaps such comparisons are already made implicitly. In fact, it may be difficult to imagine having a conscious experience in ways that does not involve such implicit comparisons. When we see red, we see it as looking rather different from blue. Red looks the way it does because it looks somewhat closer to orange, to pink, to brown, than to blue. Red looks the way it does because it looks *redder* than everything else.

We can call this a structural, relational, or holistic view of perceptual experiences. The idea is that a conscious experience cannot really be defined in isolation. If a creature is only ever to see a single flash of light in its entire life and evolutionary history, there is perhaps just no fact of the matter whether the flash will look red or green. It will just look like an indistinct, nondescript flash—if it looks like anything at all. The qualitative experience of seeing specific colors only comes about because there are different colors that we can see and subjectively distinguish from each other.

This view has been well-articulated by philosophers. In recent years, authors like Austen Clark (2000) and David Rosenthal (2010) have developed detailed versions of this line of thinking. The central idea is that we can determine the qualitative character of an experience based on the position of the relevant stimulus on a *mental quality space*. Such a space is a theoretical posit, construed such that stimuli that are subjectively similar are placed close to each other on the space. In other words, each point on the space represents a stimulus, and the distance between two points reflects the discriminability between two stimuli.

Note that this pairwise discriminability here is defined functionally, as in psychophysics. So two stimuli are more discriminable from each other if the subject is more able to distinguish them behaviorally. As such, the quality space allows us to characterize the subjective quality of conscious experiences in functional terms, without circularity. The distinctive phenomenal quality in consciously perceiving a stimulus is determined by how that stimulus is functionally distinguishable from other stimuli for the subject (Figure 9.1).

In the chapter I will flesh out how this mental quality space view fits well with the theory of perceptual reality monitoring (PRM) introduced in Chapter 7. So taken together we have an empirically grounded theory of consciousness that can account for the phenomenal character of subjective experience too.

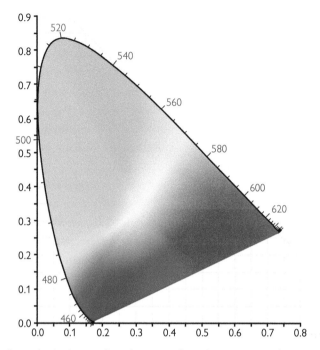

Figure 9.1 A hypothetical mental quality space for color perception for a particular individual; the distance between two points here concerns the individual's ability to distinguish between the two stimuli, rather than the objective physical similarity between the stimuli, so this space is different for different individuals. The subjective similarity between two colors can be explained by the degree of overlap between the relevant neuronal coalitions. Colors represented by more distinct populations are functionally easier to be distinguished.

9.3 "Knowing" the Quality Space

Given that we *know* what it is like to have a certain conscious experience, we presumably represent the relevant information in our brains somehow. But just because the qualitative or phenomenal character of subjective experience is best described relationally, it does not mean that we have to do it in terms of the positions on a quality space. As I have done above, we can also do it in propositional forms (i.e., something like sentences: seeing red is somewhat like orange, a little like pink, or brown, nothing like blue, nothing like silver, *and so on*).

But to *exactly* spell out the full proposition including all the relevant relations with *all the possible stimuli* would be way too clumsy, to the point that it is virtually impossible. Perhaps this explains why the quality of subjective experience seems so hard to articulate; philosophers sometimes say that it is just *ineffable*. Representing this subjective quality in terms of the location of a space is a handy alternative. It encapsulates a lot of information conveniently. But such spatio-geometrical information is only useful if we have some grasp of that space. It's no good to talk about a coordinate on a map if we don't even know what the map is.

How do we represent the mental quality space? This may seem rather challenging. The space allows for all the possible stimuli that one can perceive. Furthermore, one needs to know the discriminability of *any* two stimuli. Because the discriminability concerns how well oneself can perform the discrimination, that's a lot of self-knowledge involved.

Fortunately, there may be a plausible shortcut. The behavioral discriminability between two stimuli ultimately comes from the neural representations themselves. Suppose two colors activate very similar patterns of neural activity. Let's say for the neurons excited by these two colors, 98% of them fire at similar levels for both. By just knowing this fact, the brain should be able to infer that the two colors are not very discriminable. On the other hand, if there is a third stimulus that activates an entirely different neuronal population, the brain should "know" that it should be very discriminable from the two colors. The difficulty in behaviorally distinguishing two stimuli comes from the fact that the relevant sensory neural codes are similar. Therefore, if the brain "knows" what stimuli are represented by certain activity patterns, it should be able to tell how discriminable the stimuli are, by comparing the corresponding activity patterns.

Of course, here I put the word *know* in quotes, meaning that I use it in a subpersonal, implicit sense. The prefrontal cortex is not a person, and if it "knows" something, it does not mean that the person having that prefrontal cortex knows it explicitly. It may not be something that we can articulate easily without further reflections. But the information is there. It is implicitly known.

Recall that according to PRM, a specific higher-order mechanism (akin to a discriminator in generative adversarial networks (GANs) discussed in Chapter 6) determines whether some sensory activity should give rise to subjective experience. The mechanism *refers* to first-order sensory states, in a way that was likened to using indexes or addresses (Section 7.6). But what are these addresses? In the mammalian brain, sensory neuronal representations are spatially laid out. Different sensory representations are often supported by different neurons, sometimes in distinct brain regions, rather than by different firing patterns within the same set of neurons. This is why in Chapter 3 Section 3.11 we likened the sensory cortices to a piano.

For the prefrontal cortex to be able to target specific first-order states, for the purpose of attention, cognitive control, etc., it must "know" this spatial layout of sensory neurons somehow. It needs to "know" where the top-down signals should go. But once this layout is "known," one can already infer the discriminability between two stimuli fairly easily, at least by approximation. A pair of stimuli are not so discriminable if their spatial addresses are very similar.

An analogy may help: suppose I tell you that there are two words I'm concerned with, and they are both on page 148 of the *Oxford English Dictionary*. By giving you these rough "addresses" (the page number), you can already guess that the two words are quite likely to start with the same letter. In fact, if you know the dictionary well, you may even know exactly what that letter is. And then I can be more precise about the address: let's say one word is at line 12 of the first column, and the other word is at line 15 of the same column. Given that, one can infer that the two words likely share the first few letters. They may even look similar at a glance. All of this can be derived because we know how the dictionary is organized.

So similarly, I argue that higher-order mechanisms in the prefrontal cortex also implicitly "know" the mental quality space, at least approximately. That is because they have to "know" the spatial organization of the sensory neurons, as well as what these neurons represent, in order to allow the relevant *top-down* processes to function. When the perceptual reality monitor "decides" that some neurons representing color red are correctly representing the world right now, by *referring* to these neurons correctly, the mechanism already has the information that the color is nothing like blue or silver. It may be somewhat more like brown, orange, or pink, or maybe purple. But definitely nothing like the taste of vanilla ice cream—at least for me.

9.4 Metacognitive Benefits

The last point about vanilla ice cream is perhaps more than just a silly remark. It may indeed depend on the person. To me, color red is just nothing like ice cream of any flavor at all. But some may feel it is somewhat more like the taste of strawberry ice cream rather than chocolate ice cream. This sort of thing is ultimately somewhat subjective. Some people are more imaginative than others. Yet others experience atypically strong links between stimuli from different sensory modalities—a condition known as synesthesia (Baron-Cohen and Harrison 1997).

Going back to colors, two patches of red may also be more distinguishable for some people than others. Some people may think crimson and scarlet are clearly distinct. In a formal psychophysical test they may do well even at very brief presentations, followed by a mask, for example. Someone like myself may be rather poor at doing that.

This is to say, there are considerable individual differences in how experiences may be subjectively similar to one another, as measured by one's ability to distinguish between them in pairwise comparisons. So, for the higher-order mechanisms to implicitly represent the mental quality space, rich metacognitive information specifically *about oneself* has to be encapsulated. We can unpack this a bit by thinking explicitly about the mental quality space too.

Suppose we have the space laid out in front of us, as in Figure 9.1. This is not to be confused with the typical color space, defined in terms of physical dimensions such as *hue*, *saturation*, and *brightness*. This is a space specific to each person, based on the individual's neural codes, or the ability to distinguish between any two stimuli in the space. Suppose I quickly flash a color patch to the subject and ask if it was crimson or scarlet. Let's say the subject sees the patch as closer to crimson rather than scarlet, and answers accordingly. How confident should the subject be? Regarding this, the mental quality space contains very useful information. If crimson is very far from scarlet, the person should feel more confident. Likewise, based on the space, the person should know that a two-choice discrimination between scarlet and blue would be easier still *because* blue is so far away on the mental quality space.

Perhaps this accounts for why the mechanisms for PRM are also involved in metacognition too (Sections 5.9, 6.8–6.9, and 7.5), at least in part. That is to say, to "know" the mental quality space is to have some kind of metacognitive, self-knowledge.

9.5 Analog Representations

The discussion in Section 9.4 depends critically on the assumption that two stimuli are more easily confused with one another when the relevant neural activity patterns share similar spatial addresses. For a neural pattern, if we add a small amount of neuronal noise to it, the percept should not change very much. The result should be quite similar to the original percept. A radical change in content is only possible if we change the neural activity pattern to a larger degree.

This point may sound so trivial that it just seems tautological. But in fact, this is only true of pictorial or analog representations. For symbolic or sentence-like representations when you change just a single letter in a sentence sometimes the entire message changes. For example, "I will pay my landlord in time" versus "I will play my landlord in time."

So what are analog or pictorial representations exactly? There are very many definitions, concerning distinct key features of these representations (Beck 2015). But for our purposes, it suffices to focus on the issue of noise tolerance described in the preceding paragraphs. We can say that analog representations tolerate noise more gracefully, as compared to symbolic or sentence-like representations. And then we can say that pictorial representations are a particular type of analog representations, where the content more gracefully tolerates *spatial* noise—that is, noise that changes the spatial properties of the physical representations. For example, if a neuronal firing pattern shifts spatially to a neighboring location of very close proximity, we often expect the content not to change so drastically, as compared to moving the same firing pattern to another group of neurons many synapses away in the cortex. In this sense, the sensory codes in the mammalian brains are both pictorial and analog. (Sometimes I will say that pictorial representations are spatially analog.)

Recall that according to PRM, consciousness is in a sense the interface between perception and cognition. It selects the deserving first-order states for direct impact on higher-cognitive processing at the symbolic level. On this level, thoughts and beliefs are expressed in formats somewhat akin to sentences. As such, noisy sensory inputs are better filtered out, as they may cause dramatic and unpredictable errors on this higher level—they can cause multiplicative errors. Real percepts and our own imagination must be also delineated clearly as such early on, as they have vastly different implications for reasoning.

Despite the discussion in Chapter 8, some local theorists will remain skeptical that subjective experiences have anything to do with this kind of higher-cognitive reasoning. Perhaps this type of processing reminds them too much of good old-fashioned Artificial Intelligence. These symbolic-level rule-based operations may make some impressive chatbots. But it is not clear what it has to do with the real issue here: something so "raw" as *what it is like* to have certain conscious experiences.

But PRM does not say that consciousness happens *at* that higher-cognitive level. The point is just to highlight the possible causal connections, in order to avoid prematurely writing them off from the outset. Like local theorists and biopsychists (Chapter 6 Section 6.6), we too think the first-order states are important. In fact, I would go so far to agree that not only is the content of these states important, the nature of the physical representations themselves probably also matters (at least in most cases).

But as scientists, why would we stop at this realization? We wouldn't just identify these first-order states as the brute "correlates" of consciousness, as if no more can be said about them. Instead, we should understand what makes these states so special. Perhaps they are only "special" because they are functionally unlike sentences or symbolic representations. Perhaps they are "special" only because of their known anatomical and physiological properties. That is, because of their analog nature, and the way these first-order states are spatially organized in the sensory cortices, a high-order mechanism capable of "addressing" specific first-order states also contains the statistical information needed to tell what these states are *like*.

9.6 Revisiting Labeled Lines & Sparse Codes

It may not be so surprising that neural coding in the brain is mostly analog. The basic signal a neuron sends to other neurons, the action potential, or "spike," may seem like an on/off signal. It either happens or it doesn't. But typically, a single spike doesn't mean much. It's the spike rate or pattern that matters (Ainsworth et al. 2012). These are in turn rather analog-like: small fluctuations lead to small changes in content. And neuronal firing does fluctuate a lot. So, being analog may be a nice feature.

This analog nature applies to pretty much all neurons throughout the brain. But it is specifically in the sensory cortices that we find this highly spatially organized layout, where the content of a representation can be easily identified with a neuronal "address." Take the mammalian primary visual cortex for example (Tusa, Palmer, and Rosenquist 1978; Tootell et al. 1988; Engel, Glover, and Wandell 1997). The retinotopic organization means that for any two neurons, if they are close to each other in cortical space, the retinal locations for which stimulation would trigger their firing (i.e., the receptive fields of the neurons) are also more likely to be close to each other. Correspondingly, it means a small change in the spatial neuronal address should lead to a small change in the spatial content of the relevant percept.

Importantly, the coding of sensory neurons also seems relatively specific (Rose and Blakemore 1974; Hubel, Wiesel, and Stryker 1978; Tootell et al. 1988; Ben-Yishai, Bar-Or, and Sompolinsky 1995). For a neuron in the early visual cortex, the receptive field is often just a fraction of the entire retinal space; it seems to mainly "care" about stimuli placed with a small spatial location on the retina. Featural tuning is likewise often narrow. For a neuron, it may only care about line segments of a particular (narrow range of) orientation. It may not respond to motion, color, or sound, for example. Recall from Chapter 3 Section 3.11, sometimes we say that neurons are like "labeled lines" (Gross 2002), as in a neuron can be given a label indicating what it signals: "cats presented in this spatial location," or "45-degree right-tilted lines in that spatial location." With respect to the qualitative content, it is as if this spatially specific label is all that really matters. For the same neurons, increase in firing often just indicates that the luminance contrast increases; the signal is stronger. To change the content qualitatively, we need to activate different neurons. And often, the further away the neurons are, the more different is the resulting content.

Very much related to the concept of "labeled lines," sensory neurons are also sometimes said to adopt a "sparse" code (Olshausen and Field 2004). This means that at a given time, only very few neurons are involved in signaling the presence of a specific stimulus; most other neurons just firing at baseline level. Again, this means that there is a very clear spatial layout. To tell what the stimulus is, one only needs to know which neurons are active—or in other words, "where" is the activity.

That is why so much information can be read out or "decoded" from the fine-grained voxel patterns in functional magnetic resonance imaging (fMRI), especially within the sensory cortices, even though the signals measured are sluggish, reflecting minimal neuronal dynamics. This is also one of main reasons why decoding information from the prefrontal cortex is hard, leading some authors to mistakenly think of fMRI or electroencephalogram activity there as not reflecting specific content. Such methodological difficulty is just as expected because coding in the prefrontal cortex is known to be far less sparse (Rigotti et al. 2013; Fusi, Miller, and Rigotti 2016; Lindsay et al. 2017).

9.7 Fruit Flies

One may argue that vision, like hearing, is intrinsically spatial. Perhaps that's why neural coding is spatial for these modalities? When we see or hear a stimulus, we typically know where it comes from, or where it falls within our sensory space. Do the principles discussed in Section 9.6 apply also to sensory modalities like olfaction? Turns out, there is likewise a similar sparse coding scheme (Vosshall, Wong, and Axel 2000).

In particular, in the well-studied fruit fly olfactory system, there seems to be an active mechanism of *sparsification*. That is, at the sensory receptor level, there are just about 50 types of receptors. Together they form a combinatorial "dense" code—as in the opposite of "sparse," meaning that one single odor may activate many types of receptors, to varying degrees. But the receptors are projected (somewhat randomly) to roughly as many as 2000 Kenyon cells in the mushroom body. Feedback from a later stage of processing means that all but the top 5% of Kenyon cells with the highest-firing are suppressed. This results in a very sparse code at the Kenyon cells level, as if by "design."

What's the advantage of this kind of sparse coding scheme? Computer scientists have been inspired by how common this architecture is in the nervous system, and found that this helps to solve some challenging real-world computational problems. For example, with this sparse code, similar odors are often represented by common Kenyon cells, at least partially. Because only a few Kenyon cells are activated for a specific odor, any overlap in the Kenyon cell's firing pattern between two odors means that the two odors are likely similar, or possibly the same. It was suggested that this can help to overcome the challenging problem of *similarity search*. That is, given an odor, it may be useful to find out what other odors are similar. This can, for example, help us make generalizations for learning; similar odors may represent similar food values. Interestingly, a formal analysis shows that a computational architecture akin to the fruit flies olfactory sparse code system can outperform previous algorithms invented by computer scientists (Dasgupta, Stevens, and Navlakha 2017).

Another study showed that this scheme of sparsified coding can help an agent determine whether a stimulus is novel, that is, not having been encountered before (Dasgupta et al. 2018). Again, formal analysis shows that the sparsified coding scheme found in fruit flies can perform better than previous computer algorithms.

The reader may wonder if this means that the humble fruit fly is conscious, in the sense of knowing what an odor is subjectively *like*. The answer, at least according to PRM, is probably not. It is unclear if fruit flies have perceptual reality monitors (i.e., discriminators in a GANs-like framework). The view put forward here is not that just having analog or pictorial sensory representations is enough for consciousness. Having these representations allow subjective experiences to *potentially* occur with their distinct qualitative characters. But subjective experiences arise *only* when these representations are appropriately addressed by a perceptual reality monitor "knowing" the spatial layout of these addresses.

Also, although the Kenyon cells in fruit flies show sparse coding, the spatial organization may seem to be not as systematic or structured as in the human sensory cortices. At a first glance, the projections from the olfactory receptors to the Kenyon cells look totally random. That is rather unlike the situation in the mammalian visual and auditory cortices, where a clear and systematic spatial structure is preserved.

This lack of distinct spatial structure in coding in specific stages of olfactory processing is not just in the fruit flies, but present also in mammals (Kay 2011). However, we should distinguish between representations that are *physically* spatial analog, and representations that are *functionally* spatial analog. Olfactory coding may not show a clear spatial organization from the perspective of an experimenter holding a microscope. But functionally, it could be fundamentally similar to coding in the mammalian visual system. That is to say, let's say we hypothetically scramble around the neurons in the visual system of a mammal, while keeping the connections between the neurons the same. This should not fundamentally change the basic computational properties of the circuit. It would just muddle physical structure from an external perspective. But functionally, the internal analog structure is determined by how things are wired, which would remain just the same.

So, we can think of the olfactory system as just being physically scrambled. But functionally, the same spatial analog structure is known to exist; similar odors share similar neuronal codes (Endo, Tsuchimoto, and Kazama 2020; Pashkovski et al. 2020). To the extent that both olfaction and vision give rise to qualitative experiences in humans—there is something it is like to smell as much as to see—it seems that what is really important is this *functional* aspect of the spatial analog nature of representations. In neural network models, we sometimes call this representational property "smoothness" (Jin et al. 2020; Rosca et al. 2020).

9.8 Mantis Shrimps

To drive home the point that it is functions rather than sheer physical spatial layout that is really essential, let's consider the example of color vision in the mantis shrimp (Thoen et al. 2014). These crustaceans have over a dozen photoreceptor types, many more than we do. Surprisingly, however, mantis shrimps are not very good at fine-grained color discrimination. That is not because the photoreceptors themselves lack precision. Rather, it has more to do with the ways things are wired up the nervous system. In humans and other mammals capable of color vision, signals from the different photoreceptors are mixed together in an "opponency" scheme, meaning that it is often the relative difference in activation levels between the signaling channels that really matters (Schiller, Logothetis, and Charles 1990). However, in the mantis shrimp, it is as if each photoreceptor type has its own signaling channel, behaving rather independently from the others. Therefore, the mantis shrimp may be able to recognize individual colors detected by the different photoreceptor types. But these receptors don't coordinate together to form a continuous spectrum for fine-grained discrimination.

In other words, we can think of the color vision system in the mantis shrimp as having an extreme "labeled line" structure. Importantly, these labeled lines are relatively independent. A sensory neuron mainly takes input just from one type of photoreceptor and is therefore clear what color wavelength it signals. So in a sense, there is a spatial addressing system too. But it is not a pictorial system. It is not *spatially* analog. If anything, it is spatially discrete and symbolic. Different neurons just signal different color wavelengths, and they don't together form a continuous population code like we do in the human brain.

As such, it is reasonable to expect that when a mantis shrimp detects a color, it cannot tell how subjectively similar it is to the other colors that it can also detect with other photoreceptor channels. There are just different colors. The mantis shrimp cannot (in principle) spontaneously come up with another color similar to the detected one. And to the extent the colors represented by all photoreceptor types have been detected before, the mantis shrimp cannot ever detect a new color and consider it novel. The colors signaled by the number of receptor type channels are all that a mantis shrimp can detect. It does not have the architecture to represent and recognize a new "mix" of the fundamental signals, as a new color.

Together with the example of the olfactory system in fruit flies, hopefully this helps to make the contrast, to indicate what is special about our sensory cortex. Its physical structure generally matters for consciousness. But it only matters for computational reasons: it affords a *functionally* spatial analog (i.e., "smooth" and pictorial) address system. There is no magical "biopsychic" force involved.

9.9 Putting It All Together

In summary, according to PRM, we become aware of the content of a certain first-order (sensory) representation, when a discriminator-like mechanism "decides" that this content is suitable for further downstream cognitive processing (Chapter 7). If it is decided that the first-order activity probably reflects noise, the information will not be actively routed anywhere further. There will be no corresponding subjective experience. Otherwise, depending on whether the first-order information is deemed to reflect the state of the world right now, or some memory of the past, or some imagination of the future, and the like, it would be routed for making an appropriate impact on high-level cognition correspondingly. Global broadcast is one *potential* downstream consequence, which would facilitate some degree of cognitive control. But more important is that the information will be routed for making an appropriate impact on a narrative system capable of causal reasoning. Information processing at this level is symbolic rather than analog. This is one reason why unreliable, noisy signals are best filtered out early.

In Chapter 8, we did not speculate in detail what may be the brain mechanisms for this putative narrative system. Some preliminary evidence suggests that specific areas of the prefrontal cortex may be involved (LeDoux and Lau 2020), but the hippocampus is likely also important. The hippocampus contains cognitive maps (Tolman 1948; O'keefe and Nadel 1978), and is important for autobiographical, episodic memories (Tulving and Markowitsch 1998; Burgess, Maguire, and O'Keefe 2002). The interaction between the prefrontal cortex and the hippocampus is known to be important for the encoding of episodic memories (Eichenbaum 2017).

Whereas the specific regions in the sensory cortices represent various perceptual features, in a subjective memory episode, these different features need to be organized coherently together in terms of spatial and temporal references. The prefrontal and parietal cortices are closely connected, and both seem to be involved in spatial and temporal processing (Bueti and Walsh 2009; Peer et al. 2015; Marcos and Genovesio 2017). But the determination of temporal context likely depends more critically on the prefrontal circuits (Knight and Grabowecky 2000). To the extent that the prefrontal cortex is involved in spatial processing too, it probably more directly supports spatial processing with an egocentric (i.e., self-oriented) rather than an allocentric (i.e., world-oriented) frame of reference (Kesner, Farnsworth, and DiMattia 1989; Ma, Tian, and Wilson 2003). In generating our own self-narratives, it is important to distinguish between what is here and now, and the past or the future, from the point of view of oneself.

In other words, the various different brain regions likely work in concert in support of autobiographical, subjective narrative processing. Within the hippocampus, it is known that the storage of long-term memories does not take the form of a frame-by-frame detailed video-like recording. Instead, one enduring idea is that some kind of index system is used for efficient storage (Teyler and Rudy 2007; Tanaka and McHugh 2018). With these indexes one can retrieve the sensory details from the representations throughout the cortex. This suggests that the "addressing" system proposed earlier for the prefrontal mechanisms to refer to early sensory activity may not be unique.

Perhaps it makes sense for downstream areas to all refer to these same addresses or indexes when they communicate with each other about the relevant sensory content.

For an analogy, this is a bit like the way we pass hyperlinks for internet webpages in emails, without duplicating the detailed content—except that here the "hyperlinks" themselves are structured enough that we know similar links will take us to subjectively similar contents.

In a sense, this means that the different downstream brain regions communicate with an internal phenomenal "language": When the prefrontal cortex signals to the hippocampus that "this" sensory activity reflects the state of the world right now, the hippocampus "knows" that what should be encoded into our narratives is a sensory stimulus that *looks like* something, and yet unlike something else, for example. This may be how the qualitative nature of subjective experience comes about. The primary function of reality monitoring is for routing sensory information, to direct such information toward appropriate downstream symbolic-level processing. But, in doing so, the system implicitly knows what the stimulus in question is subjectively *like*. Because this "knowledge" is implicit, it may be difficult for the subject to articulate it. But it is part of the language through which our different brain mechanisms communicate.

Overall, this extended version of PRM is congruent with what we speculated back in Chapter 5 Section 5.11, about the functions of consciousness. In blindsight, or other forms of nonconscious perception, one should expect certain functions to be either impossible, or at least frequently compromised. That's because when a perceptual process does not lead to subjective qualitative experiences, chances are that the PRM is missing or malfunctioning, or it somehow does not address the relevant perceptual signal as correctly reflecting the state of the world right now. This would imply compromised spontaneous belief formation, and/or metacognition. It is unlikely that later on one would recall the experience vividly from memory. If the PRM is generally compromised *because* the overall prefrontal mechanisms responsible for top-down addressing of sensory signals are malfunctioning, we expect deficits in sensory inhibition and attention too. Alternatively, it could be that the PRM is doing fine, but the perceptual signals are themselves not spatially analog in nature. In that case one would be conscious of the relevant information in the sense of having access, but the relevant "experience" would not be qualitative. Accordingly, these signals would not support the ways our brains perform efficient similarity searches, and novelty detection. So, according to the PRM theory, full-blown qualitative consciousness is causally associated with these specific functions.

9.10 Robot Consciousness Revisited

We can flesh out the implications of this functional account in terms of a concrete example. Let us consider again the Hard Enough Problem (Section 7.13). If the analysis is correct so far, all the ingredients needed for subjective qualitative experience to occur can be simulated in artificial computational systems.

So let us think about the simple robot introduced in Section 7.13 again. Let us equip the robot with smooth, pictorial representations similar to ours on the first-order level. So now when a false alarm occurs at the "bodily damage" sensor located at a fingertip, not only will the robot find that disturbing to its ongoing cognitive reasoning. Not only will there be this stubborn assertoric force, that something is wrong at the fingertip even when all evidence suggests otherwise, the robot will also be able to think about what this sensory state is *like*—it can think about, from its own point of view, what other sensory states are similar to this state, so much so that oneself may mistake those other states as the current state. For example, the current state may be virtually indistinguishable from a similar signal in an adjacent sensor, but it is different from signals coming from another fingertip. The signals from another set of sensors detecting high pressure often co-activate with the current signal, and at high pressure intensity these signals can be confused with one another. But the current signal is nothing like gentle strokes, which are detected by another set of sensors giving very distinct signals. The robot will know all this through "introspection" alone.

Suppose the robot has cameras supporting visual capacities similar to ours too. If we ask the robot what red is like, it may reply that it is somewhat like brown, a bit like purple, pink, but nothing like blue. In particular the robot will not be answering this as if it is a general knowledge question, about the physical similarity between colors. It will answer based on how these other colors may be mistaken as red under suboptimal conditions, by its own cameras and visual processing. It can tell you whether scarlet is more like cherry or crimson, as they are sensed from its own point of view, at the current moment.

Also, when presented with a stimulus that it hasn't seen before, it will spontaneously report: "Wow I haven't seen this before." When asked to describe what it is like, it may say "It is a color patch. Something like right between red and yellow. Probably this is what other people call 'orange.'"

Can we imagine a blindsight patient ever behaving like this? If not, are we really so fundamentally different from this robot?

Ultimately, some may still find it hard to accept that this robot has anything like our subjective experiences. Intuitions vary from person to person. But are we at least somewhat on the right track, or not even close? To the die-hard skeptics, perhaps we should be reminded that our intuitions about the nature of consciousness may well turn out to be illusory—it's not that we can be mistaken about the very existence of consciousness in any form, but we may well grossly mischaracterize its fundamental nature (Frankish 2016). And importantly, remember that the Hard Enough Problem is a relative matter. What more plausible alternatives do we have? An inactive set of logic gates? A piece of brain tissue on a petri dish? A simple network capable of global broadcast?

This is not a book of philosophy, and I'm not a philosopher. But varieties of the structural-relational view have been defended in detail elsewhere, against classic philosophical challenges (Clark 2000; Rosenthal 2010). As in philosophical discussions, the debates continue. Some will always insist that there are unresolved issues, and they may not be entirely wrong about that. But the question remains: what are the alternatives? Are these alternatives going to lead to more meaningful progress?

9.11 Metaphysical Alternatives

Authors who insist that a functional account will never be satisfactory sometimes look for what they call "fundamental" theories of consciousness. Perhaps subjective experiences can only be understood at the foundational level of physical reality.

In the introduction, Sections I.4–I.6, I have already expressed my misgivings about such "physics-centric" approaches. Not all physicists are unreasonable, of course, but in trying to derive "first principles," some researchers end up ignoring basic empirical facts about our brains and psychological functions. Typically, as one gets past the unnecessarily complicated math, what passes on as "axioms" and theoretical principles often turn out to be nothing but unexamined philosophical assumptions.

But these views have also been proposed and defended within philosophy. For example, panpsychism is the view that all physical entities are conscious in some sense (Section 6.6); either they have conscious experiences themselves or they are part of a larger entity having conscious experiences.

The last point is related to what is called the combination problem (Roelofs 2019). So, some panpsychists say that even a single photon is conscious. But the content of my consciousness reflects a relatively unified perspective, not many independent streams of experiences by very many photons, molecules, and so on. So when I become conscious, all these tiny things inside my brain, each are otherwise conscious (according to the view), must somehow combine together to form *my* consciousness. But how does the content of my consciousness relate to the experiences by these photons before they are combined into mine? How does this combination work exactly? Why doesn't everything combine together so that the entire universe may also be conscious?

To the last question, some authors actually give a positive answer (!). In turn, panpsychism has generally been harshly criticized within philosophy. However, in recent years, there are signs that the view is gaining popularity; much effort has been put in to promote the view to the general public. Although scientists generally dismiss the view, some authors try to make it sound like that the view is being taken seriously by (some) neuroscientists.

There are indeed a few influential authors who take such views. But the nature of this topic of inquiry is that you will find all sorts of people advocating for pretty much any kind of view, however radical or improbable. Science should not be a matter of following the subjective opinions of some "influencers." We need evidence. We need logical arguments, not some highly speculative ideas hidden behind abstruse equations or populist authority.

And I'm not sure how this kind of fundamental theory can account for why consciousness matters at all. When I have a conscious experience, I can think and talk about what it is like. When I am in pain, I tend to really want to get rid of it. Just how does some fundamental property of some physical matter account for these functional and behavioral facts? And then there are all those issues mentioned in Chapter 8. A theory of consciousness does not necessarily have to give a detailed account of these higher-cognitive aspects of the mind and rationality. But the problem here is that it is not clear what these fundamental theories can meaningfully say, even in principle, about any such possible connections.

In fact, even for the Hard Problem itself, it's just as unclear if these theories help very much. Just how does stipulating that photons or the entire universe are conscious help to explain consciousness *as we know it*? Even if photons were conscious, supposedly their "experiences" aren't anything like the redness of red, the smell of roses, the sharp pain in a finger, for example.

And even if photons are conscious, just *why* are they so? Can we not imagine a universe in which photons are *not* conscious? So even if they were indeed conscious, are we to accept this as just a brute fact? Why isn't it just as plausible a brute fact that creatures who truthfully think they are conscious are, and photons just aren't?

9.12 End Game?

The last questions I raised in Section 9.11 are unlikely to discourage philosophers holding panpsychist views. To some of them, perhaps their version of brute fact—that everything is somewhat conscious just because that's the way it is—is just somehow more elegant and parsimonious than whatever else we intuitively think. But as in physics, we have also seen how a dogmatic preference of subjective theoretical beauty has led science astray (Hossenfelder 2018).

Amid all the heady metaphysical speculations, it may also be easy to forget why society values science as such. As Richard Feynman famously said, "science is like sex: sometimes something useful comes out, but that is not the reason we are doing it" (Feynman and Leighton 2001). But given all the unresolved issues discussed in the last chapter, sometimes I do wonder: What exactly are we doing here, as a discipline? It may be all good and noble for one to pursue scientific "truths" for their own sake, but our answers to questions as weighty as consciousness will inevitably have practical and ethical consequences. Far from being oblivious to the issues, panpsychists often themselves discuss these potential ethical consequences. It should not be controversial that we owe it to more than our own aesthetics and scholarly ambitions to get things right.

In this context, the following quote may be telling. In defending another metaphysical view, idealism (according to which physical things don't really ever exist outside of our mental lives), Dave Chalmers (2019) wrote: "I do not claim that idealism is plausible. *No position on the mind–body problem is plausible* ... So even though idealism is implausible, there is a non-negligible probability that it is true" (italics mine).

In a way, I agree: there is indeed some non-zero probability, for pretty much anything. But overemphasizing this seems to go against the general spirit of science in practice. Scientists learn to live with imperfect theories. They say all theories are wrong, but some are more useful than others. We sometimes call these "working hypotheses" in order not to commit ourselves to thinking that they are absolutely right or complete. We should ever be open to other possibilities. But we don't invoke and promote more radical views just because the current views aren't perceived to be perfect—unless the said radical views have clear advantages over the more boring, default views.

Perhaps this difference between the disciplines is just as it should be. Philosophers are meant to explore relatively far-fetched ideas. They think ahead for us. It is in their interest to emphasize and defend the value of what they do for a living. And sometimes I agree with them too.

But as science progresses, we expect our views to mature. As more concrete phenomena are accurately predicted, more practical applications generated, eventually our theories should become more easily accepted. So long as we stay focused, we shall get there one day. Historically, this is how difficult problems are typically "solved" in the basic sciences. But this only works if the group of experts who evaluate and permit this progress are in some ways neutral. It may be harder to convince experts of the plausibility of an existing view if their own career interests depend on the very impression of an unresolved scientific mystery.

The last point should not be mistaken for a cynical argument. There need not be any intellectually dishonest ulterior motives on anyone's part. The aforementioned potential lack of neutrality can very well emerge at a group level, as certain types of individual academics with totally sincere dispositions are selected and promoted by the system consistently. Also, given their career status, perhaps it makes total sense *for them* to go for the most radical approach possible. And I am certainly not singling out philosophers; scientists participate in this same evaluative process too, and many also thrive in hypes rather than lasting progress. But all the same, if the development of the science of consciousness itself is hindered by this process, the Hard Problem may well perpetuate as a self-fulfilling prophecy (Lau and Michel 2019).

9.13 Coda: Science & Its Players

When I was young, I thought I would one day write a book to solve the Hard Problem. I still have not given up on the problem itself. But by now I recognize that it was a deluded idea. At the moment, the best that I can offer is summarized in this final chapter, an extended version of PRM which includes some elements of quality space theory. Little of that is original, and some readers will no doubt remain unconvinced.

But worse still, I now realize that perhaps no amount of books will ever be enough to solve the problem. To solve a problem we need to first recognize its nature. Certain problems require collective action. As Thomas Kuhn (1962) famously put it, in science, there are ultimately matters that "can never be unequivocally settled by logic and experiment alone." To deny the sociohistorical aspects of science is to "dehumanize" its players.

I joined the field when the late Francis Crick was still an active champion of the problem of consciousness. In the early 2000s up till his passing, there was a general sense of optimism and promise: theoretical progress shall be built upon the solid foundation of empirical caution. I'd like to think this book represents a small step inspired by that tradition. Much of the details given here will likely turn out to be wrong. But it may be good enough if I shall turn out to be wrong rather than not even wrong. I have to count on future researchers more capable than myself to correct my many errors.

In recent years, the direction of the field has become somewhat diffused. Scientific disagreements have become increasingly difficult to resolve with conventional methods. Some may think that recent trends like "open science" may help. But this overlooks some unique features of the field. There are often deep theoretical differences between research groups. But above all, I also suspect that the bigger problem may well be the *system* itself.

Since the 1990s, our field is unique in that media visibility matters disproportionately. It has become a perfectly viable strategy to ignore peer opinions and critics within the academic expert group. To advance one's own career and ideas, one would do just as well to focus on impressing editors and private donors, via personal connections and populist appeal. One may think these problems are common in other disciplines too. But our field is unique in how rampant they are, as standard mechanisms of scientific evaluation and open competition are stifled by the relative lack of public funding and tenure-track jobs, especially in the United States.

Our larger-than-life media presence means that when newcomers approach the topic, they often don't feel the need to consult the existing literature very carefully. To some, this is just an exciting new playground best suited for trying out something risky and "different." To be fair to them, following the literature can also be difficult, as known empirical falsehoods are often repeated in high profile journals, sometimes by "authoritative" figures. And yet, as a developing field we count on these newcomers to take our subject matter seriously.

Besides media hype, philosophical opinion has also become a significant factor influencing science funding. Of course, I value interdisciplinary exchanges highly. We need philosophers as critics, as well as their constructive conceptual analysis. But if they serve also as gatekeepers who control which scientists' views are promoted as gaining momentum in prominent venues, the balance can become problematic. Certain views favored by philosophers may be intellectually interesting, but they aren't necessarily conducive to scientific progress.

Accordingly, in the past few years alone, we have seen tens of millions of US dollars of private funding poured into the field, with a particular focus on the more "theoretically ambitious" projects. For our small field, the effects will no doubt be felt for decades to come.

As in any system, there are pros and cons. The future will tell whether these are for good or for ill. My only wish is that we recognize these deep structural issues rather than deny their existence.

I have also met highly influential colleagues who vehemently defend the ways things are currently done, over more "traditional" scientific models. The argument is that our science is intrinsically special, and, thereby, it requires unconventional methods with more open mindsets.

The reader may not be surprised that I do not agree with these colleagues. People will naturally and understandably defend the very system from which their careers have benefited. I myself have also done alright in the existing system. But to my mind, the field will ever remain "special," in not necessarily very good ways, if this is how we choose to continue to comport ourselves. To have any chance of inching toward our fabled "end game," we have to think about the institutional contexts that allow good science to happen, that allow *others* to succeed. We want the field to be represented by people who are fair. We need a literature that we can *trust*. But I shall refrain from discussing these issues more than I already have. After all, this is a book about science. I've been told many times by colleagues that, as scientists, it is better for us to *focus on the science* rather than to "politicize" it.

I have often wondered about the last point. Perhaps an analogy would be: as citizens, we should also *focus on living* and leave politics to the politicians. Again, there may be pros and cons for different approaches. But I submit: this may be the Truly Hard Problem of consciousness.

References

Ainsworth M, Lee S, Cunningham MO et al. Rates and rhythms: A synergistic view of frequency and temporal coding in neuronal networks. *Neuron* 2012;**75**:572–583.

Baron-Cohen SE, Harrison JE (eds). *Synaesthesia: Classic and Contemporary Readings.* Blackwell, 1997.

Beck J. Analogue magnitude representations: A philosophical introduction. *Br J Philos Sci* 2015;**66**:829–855.

Ben-Yishai R, Bar-Or RL, Sompolinsky H. Theory of orientation tuning in visual cortex. *Proc Natl Acad Sci U S A* 1995;**92**:3844–3848.

Bueti D, Walsh V. The parietal cortex and the representation of time, space, number and other magnitudes. *Philos Trans R Soc Lond B Biol Sci* 2009;**364**:1831–1840.

Burgess N, Maguire EA, O'Keefe J. The human hippocampus and spatial and episodic memory. *Neuron* 2002;**35**:625–641.

Chalmers D. Idealism and the mind-body problem. In: W Seager (ed), *The Routledge Handbook of Panpsychism*. Routledge, 2019; 353–373.

Clark A. *A Theory of Sentience*. Clarendon Press, 2000.

Dasgupta S, Sheehan TC, Stevens CF et al. A neural data structure for novelty detection. *Proc Natl Acad Sci U S A* 2018;**115**:13093–13098.

Dasgupta S, Stevens CF, Navlakha S. A neural algorithm for a fundamental computing problem. *Science* 2017;**358**:793–796.

Eichenbaum H. Prefrontal-hippocampal interactions in episodic memory. *Nat Rev Neurosci* 2017;**18**:547–558.

Endo K, Tsuchimoto Y, Kazama H. Synthesis of conserved odor object representations in a random, divergent-convergent network. *Neuron* 2020;**108**:367–381.e5.

Engel SA, Glover GH, Wandell BA. Retinotopic organization in human visual cortex and the spatial precision of functional MRI. *Cereb Cortex* 1997;**7**:181–192.

Feynman RP, Leighton R. *"What Do You Care What Other People Think?": Further Adventures of a Curious Character*. WW Norton & Company, 2001.

Frankish K. Illusionism as a theory of consciousness. *J Consciousness Studies* 2016;**23**:11–39.

Fusi S, Miller EK, Rigotti M. Why neurons mix: High dimensionality for higher cognition. *Curr Opin Neurobiol* 2016;**37**:66–74.

Gross CG. Genealogy of the "grandmother cell." *Neuroscientist* 2002;**8**:512–518.

Hossenfelder S. *Lost in Math: How Beauty Leads Physics Astray*. Hachette UK, 2018.

Hubel DH, Wiesel TN, Stryker MP. Anatomical demonstration of orientation columns in macaque monkey. *J Comp Neurol* 1978;**177**:361–380.

Jin P, Lu L, Tang Y et al. Quantifying the generalization error in deep learning in terms of data distribution and neural network smoothness. *Neural Netw* 2020;**130**:85–99.

Kay LM. Olfactory coding: Random scents make sense. *Curr Biol* 2011;**21**:R928–R929.

Kesner RP, Farnsworth G, DiMattia BV. Double dissociation of egocentric and allocentric space following medial prefrontal and parietal cortex lesions in the rat. *Behav Neurosci* 1989;**103**:956–961.

Knight RT, Grabowecky M. Prefrontal cortex, time and consciousness. *The New Cognitive Neurosciences*. (2nd ed), Cambridge, MA: The MIT Press, 2000; pp. 1319–1339.

Kuhn TS. *The Structure of Scientific Revolutions: 50th Anniversary Edition*. University of Chicago Press, 1962.

Lau H, Michel M. A socio-historical take on the meta-problem of consciousness. *Journal of Consciousness Studies* 2019;**26**:136–147.

LeDoux JE, Lau H. Seeing consciousness through the lens of memory. *Curr Biol* 2020;**30**:R1018–R1022.

Lindsay GW, Rigotti M, Warden MR et al. Hebbian learning in a random network captures selectivity properties of the prefrontal cortex. *Journal of Neuroscience* 2017;**37**:11021–11036.

Marcos E, Genovesio A. Interference between space and time estimations: From behavior to neurons. *Front Neurosci* 2017;**11**:631.

Ma Y-Y, Tian BP, Wilson FAW. Dissociation of egocentric and allocentric spatial processing in prefrontal cortex. *Neuroreport* 2003;**14**:1737–1741.

Nagel T. What is it like to be a bat? *Philos Rev* 1974;**83**:435–450.

O'keefe J, Nadel L. *The Hippocampus as a Cognitive Map.* Clarendon Press, 1978.

Olshausen BA, Field DJ. Sparse coding of sensory inputs. *Curr Opin Neurobiol* 2004;**14**:481–487.

Pashkovski SL, Iurilli G, Brann D et al. Structure and flexibility in cortical representations of odour space. *Nature* 2020;**583**:253–258.

Peer M, Salomon R, Goldberg I et al. Brain system for mental orientation in space, time, and person. *Proc Natl Acad Sci U S A* 2015;**112**:11072–11077.

Rigotti M, Barak O, Warden MR et al. The importance of mixed selectivity in complex cognitive tasks. *Nature* 2013;**497**:585–590.

Roelofs L. *Combining Minds: How to Think about Composite Subjectivity.* Oxford University Press, 2019.

Rosca M, Weber T, Gretton A. and Mohamed S. A case for new neural network smoothness constraints. Proceedings on "I Can't Believe It's Not Better!" at NeurIPS Workshops, in Proceedings of Machine Learning Research 2020;**137**:21–32. Available from https://proceedings.mlr.press/v137/rosca20a.html.

Rose D, Blakemore C. An analysis of orientation selectivity in the cat's visual cortex. *Exp Brain Res* 1974;**20**:1–17.

Rosenthal D. How to think about mental qualities. *Philosophical Issues* 2010;**20**:368–393.

Schiller PH, Logothetis NK, Charles ER. Role of the color-opponent and broad-band channels in vision. *Vis Neurosci* 1990;**5**:321–346.

eTanaka KZ, McHugh TJ. The hippocampal engram as a memory index. *J Exp Neurosci* 2018;**12**:1179069518815942.

Teyler TJ, Rudy JW. The hippocampal indexing theory and episodic memory: Updating the index. *Hippocampus* 2007;**17**:1158–1169.

Thoen HH, How MJ, Chiou T-H et al. A different form of color vision in mantis shrimp. *Science* 2014;**343**:411–413.

Tolman EC. Cognitive maps in rats and men. *Psychol Rev* 1948;**55**:189–208.

Tootell RB, Switkes E, Silverman MS et al. Functional anatomy of macaque striate cortex. II. Retinotopic organization. *J Neurosci* 1988;**8**:1531–1568.

Tulving E, Markowitsch HJ. Episodic and declarative memory: Role of the hippocampus. *Hippocampus* 1998;**8**:198–204.

Tusa RJ, Palmer LA, Rosenquist AC. The retinotopic organization of area 17 (striate cortex) in the cat. *J Comp Neurol* 1978;**177**:213–235.

Vosshall LB, Wong AM, Axel R. An olfactory sensory map in the fly brain. *Cell* 2000;**102**:147–159.

Index

For the benefit of digital users, indexed terms that span two pages (e.g., 52–53) may, on occasion, appear on only one of those pages.

Figures are indicated by *f* following the page number

access consciousness 19–20, 23, 29–30, 159
adaptation effects
    attention 98
    binocular rivalry 44
addressing system *see* index or addressing system
affective experiences and narratives interaction 183–85
affective learning 185–86
agency self, 22–23, 170, 180
    and emotions 165–66
    loss of sense of 180–81
amnesia 61, 145
amygdala 57–58, 165–66
analog 154, 202–4
animals 25, 26, 151, 166–67, 169–70
    intuitions 152
    no-cognition 51
    rats 64
    see also monkeys
anterior cingulate 57, 73
anterior prefrontal area 73
aphantasia 27–28, 129–30, 131–32, 160
appearance boosting 96
Aristotle 18
Artificial Intelligence 142, 167–68, 203
assertoric force 153–55, 157, 162, 164–65, 168–69, 211
association cortex 24, 57
Association of the Scientific Studies of Consciousness (ASSC) 5
associative conditioning 185
associative learning 186, 187, 190
attention 9, 83–103
    and conscious control of behavior models 4
    endogenous 117–18
    filling-in 97–99
    iconic memory 84–85
    inflation 92–94
    inflation limitations 94–97
    lesions and prefrontal cortex damage 73–74, 77
    load theory 86–87
    local theories 100–1, 132, 134
    necessity for 85–86
    overflow 89–91
    post-cuing impact on early sensory activity 87–88
    quality space 201
    representations, single versus multiple levels of 99–100
    richness of experience, apparent 88–89
    speckled hen philosophical puzzle 83
    summary statistics and peripheral vision 91–92
    see also load theory of attention
attentional blink 46–47
attentional cueing 117
attentional modulation 101

autobiographical memories 187–88, 209
autobiographical subjective narrative processing 209–10

Baar, B. 14
backfiring 89
back-up systems 118
Bayes, T. 153
behavioral measures 61–62
beliefs and reality 175–76
benefits of consciousness 107–24
    clinical applications 121–22
    decoded neurofeedback (DecNef) and threat reduction 122–21
    endogenous attention 117–18
    evolutionary outlook 107
    free will as an illusion 109
    global theories 122–24
    Impossible Situations 110–12
    inhibition and exclusion 115–16
    intuitively 'improbable' situations 118–19
    metacognition 116–17
    performance matching and statistical power 114–15
    subliminal priming experiments, limits of 112–14
    volition 107–8
bilateral lesions 60, 61
binocular rivalry 41*f*, 144
    neural correlates of consciousness (NCC) 41–43, 44, 47, 48, 50–52
    nonconscious 133
biopsychism 137–38, 139, 146, 168, 203
bistable percepts 41
blindness
    change blindness 71, 94
    functional 60
    inattentional 86, 88, 93, 94
blindsight 3–4, 9, 28, 144–45
    attention 85
    decoded neurofeedback (DecNef) 119
    global theories 130
    Hard Problem 210
    higher-order failures 164
    higher-order thought or beliefs 154
    intuitions 152
    local theories 133–35
    patient GY 45, 47, 115–16, 117–19
    and primary visual cortex (V1) 35–36
    subliminal priming 113–14
    and V1 damage 52
    see also super-blindsight
blind spot 97, 98
Block, N. 19, 50, 51, 84, 88–89, 92, 136
Bloom, P. 184

Boly, M. 61
Brickner, R.M. 61
Broca's area 60
Brown, R. 139, 151

Cannon, T.D. 182–83
Carrasco, M. 96
causal inferences 177
causal reasoning 177, 180
central foveal vision 91–92
central versus peripheral vision 93
central workspace 24
centrist position 139–40, 145, 146, 175
cerebral cortex 36
Chalmers, D. 2, 214
change blindness 71, 94
change detection task 89–90, 90f
chemical inactivations 72–73
children and infants 25, 167
Clark, A. 198
claustrum 57–58, 146
Cleeremans, A. 139
clinical applications 121–22
Cobain, K. 3
cognitive control and quality space 201
cognitive dissonance 4
coherent synthesis, necessity for 25–26
collective consciousness 179
colour vision in Mantis shrimp 207–8
coma patients and experimental confounders 21–22
combination problem 212–13
computer programs 131
conceptual memory representations 188
conditioning, associative 185
confabulations
    schizophrenia 181–82
    split-brain patients 178–79
confounders 30, 51
    see also experimental confounders; stimulus
        confounders; task-performance capacity confounders
conscious episodic recall 69–70
conscious experience: qualitative aspects 197
consciousness as purposeful control 29–30
consciousness as the state an individual is in 29–30
conscious seeing 73
content mismatch 36–39, 135–36
contrivance 135–36
Corlett, P. 163–64
corpus callosum 60, 178
correlates see neural correlates of consciousness (NCC)
Cortese, A. 141
counter-conditioning with reward 120
counterfactual reasoning 177, 184
Cowan's K 90
Cowey, A. 115–16
Craske, M. 121
Crick, F. 3, 5, 215–16
'crisis of neurology' and placebo pain 188–89
criterion artifacts 113–14
crowding 94, 101
culture 28, 182, 186

decoded neurofeedback (DecNef) 121
    benefits of consciousness 123
    fear and trauma 188
    and threat reduction 119–21
Deecke, L. 107–8

definitions 17–18
degeneracy 59–60, 77
Dehaene, S. 14, 16–17, 40–41, 47, 69, 110, 111–12, 123, 129–30
Del Cul, A. 71
delusions 163–64, 180–81, 182
Dennett, Dan 13, 99, 100
detection 77, 113, 144, 145–46
    bias 95
    change detection task 89–90, 90f
    failures 73–74
    and metacognition 140–41
    tasks 71–72
Diamond, J. 190
Dienes, Z. 112
direct stimulation 72–74, 75–76
discriminability 113
    quality space 200, 201
    structural-relational view 198
discrimination task 45, 145–46
    four-choice 90
    two-choice 72, 130
    visual 71
discriminators 142–43, 166, 167, 168–69, 208–9
    fruit fly olfactory system 206
    imagery phenomenology 160
    index, gating and richness of experience 159
    inner sense 156–57
    quality space 200
    schizophrenia 181
dispositionalist position 155
dissociation 145
    see also double dissociation
distal cause versus the 'engine' itself 39
distractor effect 116
Doerig, A. 38
dominance
    binocular rivalry 44
    performance capacity 42–43
dorsolateral prefrontal cortex 57, 59–61, 64, 71, 72, 161
double dissociation 67–68, 131–32
double-drift illusion 37, 39–40
dreams 165
    coma patients and experimental confounders 21
    fast versus slow consciousness 187
    implicit versus explicit reality monitoring 161–63
    lucid 162
Durkheim, É. 179

economics and political polarization 189–90
Edelman, G. 5
Einstein, A. 6–7
emotions 28, 166, 170, 189
    affective experiences and narratives 183, 184–85
    affective learning 185–86
    and agency 165–66
    beliefs and reality 175
    fast versus slow consciousness 187
episodic memory 4
error detection 111–12
Europe 10
event-related potentials (ERP) 46–47
P3 component 47, 49
evolutionary outlook 107
exclusion 115–16
experimental confounders 129
    and coma patients 21–22
    and purposeful behavior 22–24

exposure therapy 187–88
extrastriate areas and/or feedback projections 15, 37, 136
eye movements 99

false consciousness 179
familiarity, implicit sense of 69–70
fast (System 1) thinking system 186–87
fear and trauma 187–88
feedback processes 134
feedforward only architecture 142
feedforward processes 15, 134
Festinger, L. 4
Feynman, R. 214
filling-in and attention 97–99
first-order state 68, 154, 155, 208–9
    analog representations 203–4
    imagery phenomenology 160
    index, gating and richness of experience 157f, 158–59
    inflation 164–65
    inner sense 156, 157
    quality space 200–1
    reality monitoring and dreams 161
    robot consciousness 211
flashbacks 187–88
Fleming, S. 65, 66–68, 69, 70, 71, 74
flicker fusion 44
four-choice discrimination task 90
free will 28
as an illusion 109
Freudians 191, 192
Freud, S. 191
Frith, C. 181, 182
frontal polar cortex 57, 63, 65
fronto-parietal network 39–40, 131
fruit fly olfactory system 205–7
functional advantages of conscious processing 27
functional blindness 60
functionalism 137–38, 139, 143–44
    internal 138, 139
    long arm 137–38
functional magnetic resonance imaging (fMRI) 87, 109,
    110–11, 116, 119–20, 121, 122, 205
neural correlates of consciousness (NCC) 37–38, 39, 42,
    44, 45–46, 48–49
functional movement disorders 189
functions of consciousness 24, 26
fundamental theories of consciousness 212

Gabor patches 37, 38f, 87–88
gating mechanisms 158–59, 177–78, 182–83
Gazzaniga, M. 4
general theory of consciousness 151
generative adversarial networks (GANs) 141–43, 143f,
    156, 158, 166, 200, 206
global anesthesia 21
global broadcast 208–9
global information access 23
global neuronal workspace theory 9, 14, 110, 131
global theories 13–14, 15f, 17, 24, 25, 131–32, 144
    access consciousness versus phenomenal
        consciousness 19–20
    attention 85, 86, 88, 91, 92, 94, 102
    benefits of consciousness 122–24
    binocular rivalry 44
    centrism 139
    children and animals 25
    content mismatch in early visual areas 38

contrivance 135–36
endogenous attention 117
functions of consciousness 24, 26
Hard Enough problem 169
Impossible Situation 110, 111–12
index, gating and richness of experience 159
intuitively improbable situations 118
lesions and prefrontal cortex damage 57, 68, 69, 77
machines and robots 25
neural correlates of consciousness (NCC) 24, 25, 45–46, 51
opposing dogmas 137, 138
performance-capacity confounders 47
performance matching and statistical power 114
problems 129–31
reality monitoring and dreams 161, 162–63
reports 49
richness of subjective experience 24
stimulus confounder 40–41, 42, 52
theoretical goal posts 16–17, 29
theoretical upshot 27, 28
Gödel 2
gray zone 22

Haidt, J. 184, 189
hallucinations 36, 73, 134–35
    auditory 181, 182
    reality monitoring and dreams 161, 162
    schizophrenia 181, 182
    sensory 163–64, 180–81
    visual 164
Hard Enough Problem 168–69, 170, 211–12
Hard Problem 19, 29, 197–217
    analog representations 202–4
    beliefs and reality 175
    colour vision in Mantis shrimp 207–8
    conscious experience: qualitative aspects 197
    labeled lines and sparse codes 204–7
    metacognitive benefits 201–2
    quality space, 'knowing' 199–201, 199f
    structural-relational view 197–98
hearing 15–16
hemispatial neglect 178
here-and-now quality 27
hierarchical models 68–70, 69f, 130, 133–34
higher-order state 28, 151, 154–56
    analog representations 203, 204
    centrism 139
    failures 163–64
    Hard Problem 208–9
    imagery phenomenology 160
    impossible situation 111
    index, gating and richness of experience 157f, 158–59
    inflation 164–65
    inner sense 156, 157
    metacognitive benefits 202
    parallel versus hierarchical models 68, 70
    quality space 200–1
    reality monitoring and dreams 161, 162–63
    self, actions and responsibility 180
    see also discriminators
high-resolution perception 89–91
hippocampus 33–34, 57–58, 209–10
historical background 3–5
homophily 186
homunculus 75–76, 75f
Hume, D. 184, 189
hyperalignment 121

iconic memory 84–85
idealism 214
identity view 34
imagery
  mental 36, 161
  phenomenology 159–60
implicit versus explicit reality monitoring: dreams 161–63
Impossible Situation 110–12
inattentional blindness 86, 88, 93, 94
index or addressing system 158–59, 200–1, 204, 208, 209–10
inferior parietal region 71–72
inflation 140, 144, 164–65
  attention 92–97, 101, 102–3
inhibition 114, 115–16, 117, 118, 124, 130
  response 111, 112, 131
inner sense 156–57
insular 57–58, 165–66
intention 109
  motoric 73
introspection 211
intuitions 152–53, 189, 211–12
intuitively 'improbable' situations 118–19

Jacoby, L.L. 115–16
James, W. 96
Jastrow, J. 4

Kahneman, D. 186
Kant, I. 151
Kawato, M. 119–20
Kentridge, B. 117–18
Kenyon cells (fruit fly) 205–6
key issues 24–25
Knight, B. 61
Koizumi, A. 114, 120, 121
Koller, W.N. 182–83
Kornhuber, H.H. 107–8
Kuhn, T. 8, 215
Kwok, S. 67

labeled lines 76, 204–5, 208
Lamme, V. 15–17, 89, 134
language 14, 60, 182
Lapate, R.C. 64
lateral competition 88
lateral geniculate nucleus 101
lateral prefrontal area 63, 73, 116
Lavie, N. 102
learned threat response 120
learning 63, 65
  affective 185–86
  associative 186, 187, 190
  model-based 187
  model-free associative 187
  motor 4
  vicarious 185–86
Ledoux, J. 122
Leibniz 7
lesions and prefrontal cortex damage 57–77
  behavioral measures 61–62
  conceptual confusions about lesions 58–60
  controversial case studies 60–61
  direct stimulation 72–74
  double dissociation 67–68
  metacognition 62–64
  parallel versus hierarchical architectures 68–70

perceptual metacognition 70–72
prefrontal cortex versus rest of brain 57–58
sensory cortices 74–76
specific lesion effects 65–67
Lewy body dementia 164
Libet, B. 107–8
Liu, S. 37
load theory of attention 86–87, 88, 102
local theories 14–16, 16f, 17, 24, 25, 28, 29
  access consciousness versus phenomenal consciousness 19–20
  analog representations 203
  attention 84, 85, 86, 88–89, 91, 92, 94, 97, 100–1, 102
  beliefs and reality 175
  benefits of consciousness 123
  centrism 139
  children and animals 25
  content mismatch in early visual areas 38
  contrivance 135
  distal cause versus 'engine' 39
  functions of consciousness 24
  Hard Enough problem 169
  Impossible Situation 111
  lesions and prefrontal cortex damage 57, 73–74, 77
  machines and robots 25
  neural correlates of consciousness (NCC) 51
  opposing dogmas 136, 137–38
  performance-capacity confounders 47
  problems 132–35
  purposeful behavior and experimental confounders 23–24
  reality monitoring and dreams 161
  richness of subjective experience 24
  stimulus confounder 42
  theoretical goal posts 16, 17–201
Locke, J. 151
long-term memory 14
Luhrmann, T. 182

McCurdy, L. 65, 66–67
machines and machine consciousness 25, 26, 168, 170
  see also Artificial Intelligence; robots
Macknik, S. 15, 71
Malach, R. 15
Maniscalco, B. 63, 70, 115, 131
Mantis shrimp colour vision 207–8
Martinez-Conde, S. 15
Marxist ideas 191
masking 119
  metacontrast 45–46
  see also visual masking
matching method 95
memory 63, 65
  autobiographical 187–88, 209
  conceptual 188
  episodic 4
  iconic 84–85
  long-term 14
  metacognition 65, 66f, 66–68, 162–63
  recall, vividness of 162–63
  recognition memory tasks 182–83
  sensory memory representations 188
  visual working 155
  see also working memory
mental disorders 192
mental imagery 36, 161
mental quality space 198–201, 199f, 202, 215

'mesh' argument 89
metacognition 9, 144, 166–67
 attention 94
 benefits of consciousness 116–17, 123, 124
 and detection 140–41
 economics and political polarization 190
 endogenous attention 117
 explicit 163
 generative adversarial networks (GANs) 143
 global theories 130
 imagery phenomenology 160
 implicit and explicit 162
 inner sense 156–57
 intuitively improbable situations 118
 lesions and prefrontal cortex damage 62–64, 68, 70, 77
 nonconscious 113
 parietal cortex 131
 visual 65, 66
 see also perceptual metacognition
metacognitive benefits 201–2
metacognitive efficiency 68–69
metacognitive insight impairment 73–74
metacognitive response (confidence) 68
metacontrast masking 45–46
meta-d measure 63, 65, 66
metaphysical alternatives 212–13
metaphysical view 214
Michel, M. 38, 59, 83, 144–45
Milner, B. 4
'mindless' approach 5–6
model-based learning 187
model-free associative learning 187
modules 14
monkeys 48, 109
 lesions and prefrontal cortex damage 60, 64, 67, 71–72
 no-cognition 50
 volition 108
Morales, J. 59, 100
motion 15
motor control 14
motor cortex 33–34
motoric intention 73
motor learning 4
multivariate decoding approaches on EEG data 49
multivoxel pattern analysis (MVPA) 37, 119–20

Naccache, L. 110
narratives and narrative system 192
 affective experiences interaction 183–85
 affective learning 186
 economics and political polarization 189–90
 fast versus slow consciousness 186, 187
 narrative as 'consciousness' 179–80
 narrative level 181–82
 narratives of reality 176, 177–78
 schizophrenia 182–83
 self, actions and responsibility 180
 symbolic causal narratives 176–78
narratocracy 190
near-threshold presentation experiments 52
necessity 34–35, 85, 112–13
Neisser, U. 85–86
neural correlates of consciousness (NCC) 24, 25, 26, 136, 145, 146
 binocular rivalry 41–43, 44, 47, 48, 50–52
 blindsight patient GY 45, 47
 blindsight and primary visual cortex (V1) 35–36

content mismatch in early visual areas 36–39
 contrivance 135, 136
 correlates 33–34
 derailment 33
 distal cause versus the 'engine' itself 39
 fronto-parietal network 39–40
 global theories 45–46
 lesions and prefrontal cortex damage 57–59, 60, 77
 local theories 133
 necessity and sufficiency 34–35
 no-cognition paradigms 50–51
 performance capacity confounders 42–44, 46–48, 49, 51–52
 reports 48–49
 stimulus confounders 40–42, 49, 51
Newton, I. 7
no-cognition paradigms 50–51
no-go or stop signal 111
non-conscious/non-consciousness 122, 131–32, 145
 attention 85
 benefits of consciousness 123
 binocular rivalry 51, 133
 content mismatch in early visual areas 37
 contrivance 135
 decoded neurofeedback (DecNef) 119–20
 endogenous attention 117–18
 fast versus slow consciousness 187
 fear and trauma 188
 fronto-parietal network 40
 global theories 130
 Hard Problem 210
 higher-order thought or beliefs 154
 Impossible Situation 110–12
 information 26
 intuitions 152
 intuitively improbable situations 118
 lesions and prefrontal cortex damage 68–69
 local theories 133–34
 memories 69–70
 metacognition 116–17
 narratives as consciousness 179–80
 opposing dogmas 137–38
 optimal Bayesians and phantom pain 153, 154
 perception 145
 split-brain patients and confabulations 178
 stimuli 130
 stimulus confounder 40–41
 subliminal priming 113–14
 volition 108
 working memory 129–30
no-report paradigm 48

Odegaard, B. 61, 93
olfactory domain 71
open-head surgery 72–73
opponency scheme 207–8
opposing dogmas 136–38
optic tract 60
optimal Bayesians 153–54
orbitofrontal cortex 71, 73
overview 13–30
 access consciousness versus phenomenal consciousness 19–20
 coherent synthesis, necessity for 25–26
 coma patients and experimental confounders 21–22
 definitions 17–18
 global theories 13–14, 15*f*

overview (*cont.*)
  key issues 24–25
  local theories 14–16, 16*f*
  purposeful behavior and experimental confounders 22–24
  theoretical goal posts 16–17
  theoretical upshot 27–29
Owen, A. 22

pain
  chronic 188–89
  phantom 153–55
  placebo 188–89
Panagia, D. 190
Panagiotaropoulos, F. 50
panpsychism 136–37, 192, 212–13, 214
parallel models 68–70, 69*f*, 130, 131, 133–34, 135
parietal cortex 39–40
  benefits of consciousness 122
  binocular rivalry 44
  global theories 14, 15*f*, 46, 129, 131
  Hard Problem 209
  higher-order failures 163
  imagery phenomenology 160
  lesions and prefrontal cortex damage 59–60, 63, 69, 70, 71
  local theories 132
  neural correlates of consciousness (NCC) 24, 52
  performance-capacity confounders 47
  reality monitoring and dreams 162–63
  reports 48–49
  stimulus confounder 42
Parkinson's disease 164
Passingham, R.E. 46, 109, 145
Patient A 60–61
Patient GY and blindsight 45, 47, 115–16, 117–19
Patient HM (amnesic) 4
pattern recognition networks 142
Pavlov, I. 185
Pavlovian conditioning 187, 188
Pearl, J. 177
Penfield, W. 72–73, 75–76, 75*f*
Penrose, Sir R. 5
perception 2, 9, 28, 131–32, 138, 144, 145
  analog representations 203
  attention 83, 86, 88, 89, 90, 91, 92–93, 96, 101, 102
  bottom-up 166, 167
  colour 199*f*
  contrivance 135–36
  generative adversarial networks (GANs) 142–43
  global theories 14, 129–31
  higher-order thought or beliefs 154–55
  high-resolution 89–91
  imagery 159–60
  index and gating 158–59
  inner sense 157
  intuitions 152
  lesions and prefrontal cortex 59, 68, 70, 77
  local theories 15–16, 132, 133–34
  low-resolution 90
  neural correlates of consciousness (NCC) 40–41, 42–43, 45, 46, 47, 49, 52
  non-conscious 113–14, 145, 152, 154, 205
  optimal Bayesians and phantom pain 153
  performance matching and statistical power 114–15
  peripheral or unattended 102, 131–32, 133
  predictive coding and generative adversarial networks (GANs) 141, 142–43

self-recognized 170
stimulus confounder 40–41
subjective 52, 83, 86, 89, 114–15, 129–30, 131
subliminal priming 113–14
symbolic causal narratives 177–78
theories, higher-order 156
visual 14, 63, 69
perceptual decision-making 93, 95
perceptual experience 27–28, 198
perceptual judgment 64
perceptual load 86–87, 89
perceptual metacognition 65, 66–68, 70–72, 74, 93, 94
perceptual phenomena 95
perceptual process 19
perceptual reality monitoring (PRM) 151, 157*f*, 166, 167, 168, 170, 192
  agency and emotions 165
  analog representations 203
  beliefs and reality 175
  dreams 161, 162, 163
  fast versus slow consciousness 187
  fruit fly olfactory system 206
  Hard Enough problem 168, 169
  Hard Problem 208–9, 210, 215
  imagery phenomenology 159, 160
  implicit and explicit 163
  inflation 164–65
  metacognitive benefits 202
  quality space 200–1
  self, actions and responsibility 180
  structural-relational view 198
perceptual representation 92
perceptual rivalry 50–51
perceptual signal, internal 43
perceptual switch 41–42
performance matching and statistical power 114–15
peripheral perception 102, 131–32, 133
peripheral vision 91–92, 131–32, 140, 164, 165
Persaud, N. 45, 115–16
Peters, M. 113–14, 141
phantom pain 153–55
phenomenal consciousness 19–20, 23
phenomenal overflow 84
Phillips, I. 145
phobias 121
phonological task 110–11
physics-centric approaches 212
Pierce, C.D. 4
Pincham, H.L. 46–47
Pizarro, D.A. 184
placebo pain and the 'crisis of neurology' 188–89
political polarization and economics 189–90
post-cue procedure 84–85, 84*f*, 87–88, 89, 96, 99
posterior hot zone or posterior cortex 57–58
postperceptual thinking 51
post-traumatic stress disorders 121, 187–88
prechange identification task 90
precuneus 65, 66*f*, 67, 162–63
predictive coding 141–42, 144, 156, 166, 167
prefrontal cortex 26, 27, 28, 144, 146, 166–67
  attention 100, 101, 102
  benefits of consciousness 122
  binocular rivalry 44
  contrivance 135
  distal cause versus 'engine' 39
  endogenous attention 117
  fronto-parietal network 39–40

generative adversarial networks (GANs) 142–43
global theories 14, 15f, 45–46, 129, 130, 131
Hard Problem 209, 210
higher-order failures 163–64
higher-order thought or beliefs 154
imagery phenomenology 159, 160
Impossible Situation 110–11
inner sense 156
intuitively improbable situations 118
labeled lines and sparse codes 205
local theories 132–33, 134
metacognition and detection 140
neural correlates of consciousness (NCC) 24, 52
no-cognition 50–51
opposing dogmas 136, 138
performance-capacity confounders 47
quality space 200, 201
reality monitoring and dreams 161, 162–63
reports 48–49
schizophrenia 181
self, actions and responsibility 180
stimulus confounder 42
see also lesions and prefrontal cortex damage
presupplementary motor area 109
primary visual cortex (V1)
    attention 87–88, 101
    blindsight 35–36
    content mismatch in early visual areas 36–37
    contrivance 136
    feedback 15, 16–17
    labeled lines and sparse codes 204–5
    local theories 133, 134–35
priming approach 110–11, 112, 117, 122
    see also subliminal priming
psychogenic disorders 189
psychophysics method of adaptation 97–98
psychosis 163–64, 180–82
publication bias 39
pulvinar 146
purposeful behavior and experimental
        confounders 22–24

qualia 146
    nonfunctional 192
    pure 192

Rahnev, D. 93, 111
rational behaviour/rationality 28, 146, 175–76
readiness potential 107–8
reality and beliefs 175–76
reality monitoring
    implicit versus explicit 161–63
    see also perceptual reality monitoring (PRM)
recognition memory tasks 182–83
recurrence theory 134
recurrent activity 15, 16–17, 136
relational view of perceptual experiences 198
REM (rapid eye movement) 161, 163
repetition suppression 39
report
    confounders 57, 59
    lesions and prefrontal cortex damage 60, 73–74
    local theories 132
    neural correlates of consciousness (NCC) 48–49
    subliminal priming 113
representations, single versus multiple levels of 99–100
repulsion effect (adapted out) 97–98

repurposing 156–57
response inhibition 111, 112, 131
responsible revolutionary planning 7–8
retinopathy 75–76
richness of experience 24, 26, 27, 132, 158–59
    attention 88–89, 91, 92, 94, 96–97, 101, 102
    local theories 133
robots 25, 131, 151, 167–70, 211–12
Rosenthal, D. 139, 151, 155–56, 198
Rothwell, J. 62–63
Rounis, E. 62–63, 70, 74
Rutherford 5–6

Sasaki, Y. 119–20
Schiller, R. 190
schizophrenia 180–83
Scott, R. 112
selective looking 85–86, 88, 93
    see also inattentional blindness
self, actions and responsibility 180
self-awareness 180
self-image 187–88
self-knowledge 72
self-monitoring mechanism 180
self-organizing metarepresentational account 139
semantic task 110–11
semiconsciousness 22
sensory cortices 74–76
sensory level 181
sensory memory representations 188
sensory representation 27–28
Sergent, C. 87
Shallice, T. 4
Shibata, K. 119–20
signal detection theory 62, 63
sinusoidal gratings 37–38
Skinner, B.F. 185, 187
Skinnerian conditioning 187
Sligte 89–90, 90f, 91
slow (System 2) thinking system 176–87
Solovey, G. 93
somatosensory areas 75–76
sparse coding scheme 76, 204–7
spatial neglect 71–72
speckled hen philosophical puzzle 83, 85
Sperling, G. 84, 84f, 85, 87, 89, 96, 99
Sperry, R. 4
split-brain patients 4, 145, 178–79
statistical power and performance matching 114–15
stimulus confounders 40–42, 49, 51, 57
stroke or external trauma 60
structural view of perceptual experiences 198
Suárez-Pinilla, M. 97–98
subjective ratings and accuracy 63
subjective visibility 71, 114
subliminal instruction figure 110–11
subliminal priming 110, 123, 131
    decoded neurofeedback (DecNef) 119
    global theories 130
    limits of 112–14, 115
    local theories 134
subliminal task instruction 111
subpersonal process 28
sufficiency and neural correlates of consciousness
        (NCC) 34–35
suicidal thoughts and behavior 187–88
summary statistics and peripheral vision 91–92

super-blindsight 153
supplementary motor area 73
suppression 42–43, 44
syllogistic inference 157
symbolic causal narratives 176–78
synesthesia 201

Tascherau-Dumouchel, V. 121, 122
task demand and perception 86
task-performance capacity confounders 57, 144–45
  contrivance 135
  global theories 45, 129
  inhibition and exclusion 116
  lesions and prefrontal cortex damage 57, 65, 77
  local theories 133, 134
  metacognition 116–17
  neural correlates of consciousness (NCC) 42–44, 46–
    48, 49, 51–52
  performance matching and statistical power 114–15
  subliminal priming 114
task sets 110–11, 112
Tegmark, M. 6
temporal context effect 38
temporal duration illusions 39–40
thalamus 146
theoretical goal posts 16–17
theoretical upshot 27–29
theta-burst 62–63, 64
threat reduction and decoded neurofeedback
  (DecNef) 119–21, 122
touch 15–16
transcranial magnetic stimulation (TMS) 61–62, 63, 64,
  65, 67, 70, 71–70, 72–73, 109
trauma and fear 187–88
traumatic brain injury 21
two-choice discrimination task 72, 130

unattended background 131
unattended perception 131–32, 133
unattended periphery 99
unattended vision 140, 165
uniformity illusion 97–98, 98f, 99–100
unilateral lesions 60, 66
United States 10

Valsecchi, M. 95
van Gaal, S. 111, 134
vicarious learning 185–86
'virtual lesions' effect 36, 61–62
visibility ratings 94
vision
  central foveal 91–92
  central versus peripheral 93
  unattended 140, 165
  see also peripheral vision
visual cortex
  attention 98, 100
  binocular rivalry 44
  lesions and prefrontal cortex damage 68, 75–76, 77
  local theories 14–16, 16f, 133
  V2 visual area 87–88
  see also primary visual cortex (V1)
visual detection behavior 71
visual discrimination task performance 71
visual imagery, spontaneous 73
visual masking 40, 40f, 47, 113, 114, 129–30
visual metacognition 65, 66
visual task performance 62, 63, 71
visual working memory 155
volition 73, 107–8, 109, 165, 166, 175
Voss, U. 162

Watanabe, T. 116, 119–20
Webb, T. 143
Wegner, D. 109
Weiskrantz, L. 3–4, 52
Wokke, M. 64
working hypotheses 214
working memory 9, 131–32, 167
  attention 90–91
  benefits of consciousness 123
  generative adversarial networks (GANs) 142–43
  higher-order thought or beliefs 155–56
  Impossible Situation 111–12
  non-conscious 113, 129–30
  reality monitoring and dreams 161
workspace functions 131

Zhou, H. 37–52